# How To Study For Your FNP Certification

By Tina Shropshire FNP-C

**Copyright @Tina Shropshire. All rights reserved.**

**Disclaimers**

**Although every effort has been made to use reliable and up-to-date resources in an effort to provide accurate information, some standards may have changed as of date of publication.**

## Preface

The purpose of this text is to give the reader a short and concise quick reference guide to prepare for their FNP board certification with either the American Academy of Nurse Practitioners (AANP) or the American Nurses Credentialing Center (ANCC). The idea is for this to be a quick summary of what you will need to pass your boards the first time around without having to review every aspect of the nurse practitioner program.

Thus, the main focus of this book is to cover the topics that are actually on the exam. For example, if there are few to no questions regarding the proper way to manage a urinary tract infection (Bactrim, Cipro, or Macrobid), you won't find it in this book, although it is seen in primary care on a daily basis.

It is my mission to help the nurse practitioner profession as much as possible. If you have any suggestion as to how I can improve this text, comments, questions or concerns, please feel free to email me at tinabeanrn@hotmail.com

## About the ANCC

The exam is 200 questions of which 175 are scored and 25 are not calculated into your score. There is no way to tell the difference between the test questions, so treat each one as if it counts. There are sample test questions available and a detailed outline of the test content available on their website https://www.nursingworld.org/ancc/.

Your score will appear as either pass or fail. You can only take this exam three times within a 12-month period.

This text will focus on the clinical aspect of the exam and not go into detail about the research, theory, and policy aspects you will be expected to know for this particular exam.

## About the AANP

This exam has 150 questions on it. Only 15 questions are not scored; the other 135 questions are scored. This is a clinical exam that includes a few ethical questions. This text is designed around this exam in particular. You will need to know how to identify x-rays such as diagnosing pneumonia on an x-ray or tuberculosis. There are ecg strips included in this exam which you will need to identify.

You need a minimum score of at least 500 to pass this exam. Scores range from 200 to 800. The average pass rate is 81.6% for the exams taken in 2016 for the FNP certification.

## Table of Contents

**Cardiology**……………………………………………………..7-16

**Dermatology**…………………………………………………17-29

**ENT**……………………………………………………...30-35

**Endocrinology**……………………………………………..36-41

**Eye Disorders**……………………………………………..42-46

**GI/GU**…………………………………………………..47-54

**Hematology**……………………………………………….55-57

**ID/STD**……………………………………………………58-70

**Labs to know**………………………………………………..71

**Men's Health**……………………………………………...72-74

**Mood Disorders**……………………………………………75-76

**Musculoskeletal**……………………………………………77-83

**Neurology**……………………………………………....84-89

**Pediatrics**…………………………………………….....90-101

**Respiratory Disorders**…………………………………...102-104

**Rheumatology**……………………………………….....…105

**Women's Health**……………………………………..…106-114

**References**…………………………………………...115-133

**Abbreviations**………………………………………….134-141

# About the Author

I am a board-certified family nurse practitioner certified through the AANP. I graduated with my BSN from Oakland University in 2008 and with my MSN/FNP from University of Detroit Mercy in 2012. In preparation for my boards, I literally studied for one year before taking the exam. I studied from five popular review courses and textbooks, only to find that I was over-prepared. After paying upward of $600 for one review course, which only helped me with four exam questions, I decided to start helping future nurse practitioners prepare for the boards myself. Not only do I love studying, I love helping people conquer their fears and pass their boards the first time.

I have sat with dozens of nurse practitioner students and helped them prepare for their exam. They would ask me wild and debatable questions that are not on the exam. I would tell them to stop, breathe, and focus. If it's not on the exam, let's not worry about it.

I have taught as an adjunct faculty member at South University of Novi Michigan. When preparing my FNP students for their didactic exams, students would always want me to be extremely specific about what was on the exam. For example, if we have studied 55 topics, they wanted to know what 20 topics in particular they would need to know to pass the exam. Therefore this text is designed to be specific enough for you to pass your exam without over studying.

I have been precepting NP students since 2013. I love doing this! If you are in the Detroit area, please contact me at tinabeanrn@hotmail.com. I am booked for the rest of 2018 but have opening next year. All of my students love me, learn tons and keep in touch with me ☺

I am currently working in employee health; previous to this, I worked as a functional medicine FNP at a family practice since graduation. I am currently pursuing my DNP.

I would like to thank all the students who sat with me for one-on-one tutoring for their certification. I would like to thank my co-workers who have inspired me and my family and, most importantly, God.

Of note, most of us will not leave NP school debt free. I racked up enough student loan debt to pay for a nice size home. Recently I refinanced by student loan with Earnest. I cannot tell you how quick and easy the process was! I did everything from my phone and was approved in 3 days. I have now saved over 271 k (yes more than two hundred and fifty thousand dollars) in interested as my interest rate dropped from 7.9% to 5%. I wish I would have known about them years and years ago. I literally paid 31k in interest alone in 2017. I highly encourage you to check them out!!

https://www.earnest.com/invite/kasheena

**Click the above link and both you and I will get $200 if you decide to refinance with Earnest! You have nothing to lose** ☺

# Cardiology

## ACE INHIBITORS

Work by stopping the powerful vasoconstrictor angiotensin converting enzyme from converting to angiotensin 1 to angiotensin 2.

**What to know for the exam:** Side effects of ACE inhibitors: *CAPTOPRIL*

Cough
Angioedema
Potassium excess
Taste changes
Orthostatic hypotension
Pregnancy contraindication/Pressure drop (hypotension)
Renal failure/Rash
Indomethacin inhibition
Leukopenia (rare)

**Contraindications to ACE inhibitors:** *PARK*

Pregnancy
Allergy/Angioedema
Renal artery stenosis/Renal failure
K - hyperkalemia (potassium > 5.5)

**First line drug of choice for CHF**

**Used in patients with diabetes and HTN**

**Used in patients with diabetes and early CKD**

## A-fib/A flutter

- Atrial rates range about 250 to 320 bpm on average
- Ventricular rate is usually 120–160 bpm.
- Patient may present with heart palpitations that feel like **flip-flopping** in a patient's chest that occurs before the HR returns to a regular rate and rhythm

**What to know for the exam**: Order a Holter monitor. Know how to identify A-fib and A-flutter on an ECG strip. <u>**No p waves with A-fib!**</u> Know that patients with A-fib/A-flutter are prone to having a stroke. Your patient may also be on Coumadin with a subtherapeutic level. Know how to titrate Coumadin and digoxin depending on where your patient's INR is.

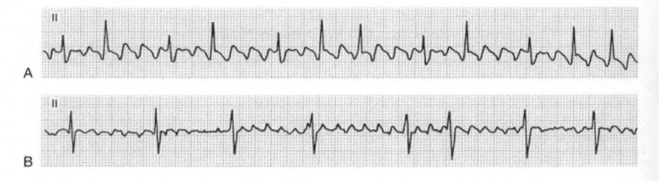

A. Atrial flutter with variable AV block
B. Course atrial fib

## Bacterial Endocarditis

- Patient who presents with a one-week history of fever, chills, musculoskeletal pain, and exhaustion; patient may have a history of MVP and a history of smoking; on physical exam, you may hear a grade 2/4 holosystolic murmur.
- Commonly seen in patients with indwelling vascular catheters, **IVDA**, and those with recent dental work completed. patient may have a murmur, peripheral emboli, retinal hemorrhages with white pale centers (Roth spots), splinter hemorrhages, or *__Janeway lesions__*

    **What to know for the exam**: Refer to ER for IV antibiotics; obtain blood cultures in the first 24 hours; signs and symptoms. **Know Janeway lesions!** (these are nontender small erythematous or hemorrhagic macular lesions on the palms or soles).

## Congestive Heart Failure (CHF)

- Patient may present with increased dyspnea, even at rest; patient usually has a long-standing h/o HTN and may have an h/o smoking
- Assess for jugular vein distention, rales, S3 gallop, ankle edema, nocturnal dyspnea or orthopnea
- Check BNP; > 400 pg/ml positive finding
- ACEI or ARB first drug of choice
- Besides ACEI, patients are usually on loop diuretics, vasodilators, and beta blockers

    **What to know for the exam:** ACEI or ARB first line drug of choice. Diagnosed with auscultation and a chest x-ray. You hear an S3 gallop with CHF, and you see jugular vein distention. **Avoid NSAIDS**, CCB, and Actos in patients with CHF.

# Cardiac Murmurs

## Literally always on the boards!

- Need to know how to grade them on a scale from 1–6, 1 being the lowest intensity and 6 being the highest intensity
- **Grade 1:** Barely audible
- **Grade 2:** Audible but soft (no intervention needed)
- **Grade 3:** Easily audible
- **Grade 4**: Easily audible with a thrill (first-time thrill is present)
- **Grade 5**: Like **Grade 4** but heard with edge of stethoscope
- **Grade 6:** Heard with stethoscope off of chest
- <u>Aortic Stenosis</u>: **Systolic** murmur with a crescendo-decrescendo pattern that radiates to the carotids; <u>this is the one murmur that would radiate to the neck</u>
- <u>Aortic Regurgitation (AR)</u>: **Diastolic** leakage of blood from the aorta.
- <u>Mitral valve prolapse</u>: Most common valvular heart condition in the US. Expect to hear a **mid-systolic click**
- **Systolic murmurs: MR AS (mitral regurgitation & aortic stenosis)**
- **Diastolic murmurs: MS AR (mitral stenosis & aortic regurgitation)**

## Coarctation of the Aorta

- Common congenital heart defect; occurs in males more often than females
- Patient may present with decreased or absent lower extremity pulses and strong upper extremity pulses
- 2D echo positive for aortic arch narrowing

- This is treated with surgical repair, stents, or balloon dilation
- Typically found in early childhood

**What to know for the exam**: Presentation

## Hyperlipidemia

- Total cholesterol >240. 200–239 considered borderline dyslipidemia; LDL > 100, HDL < 40 in men and < 50 in women
- **Statins drug of choice for lowering LDLs**
- Average risk patients need to be screening starting at age 20 and then every five years with fasting lipid panel
- Screening varies for patients with CVD risk such as HTN, DM, and family history of CVD
- **Lifestyle changes are recommended in all patients**
- Fibric acid medications (fibrates) such as fenofibrate can be taken in addition to statins but only in those with mixed dyslipidemia to control total cholesterol and triglycerides; never give gemfibrozil (fibrate) with a statin. Fenofibrate and fenofibric acid are the drugs to choose when combined a fibrate with a statin.

## Hypertriglyceridemia

- Fasting lipids are considered optimal < 150
- Borderline 150–190
- Hypertriglyceridemia 200–499 & > 500 is considered severe and puts patients at risk for pancreatitis
- More common in patients with obesity, DM or pre-DM, and CAD
- Lifestyle changes cannot be overstated
- Medication treatment is based on age and other CVD risk but includes moderate to high intensity statin with lifestyle changes

- If levels are > 500 fibric acid medications such as gemfibrozil or fenofibrate micronized pills are indicated with lifestyle changes

## NIACIN

- Niacin helps improve a patient's HDLs and triglycerides
- Vitamin B3
- Use 1500 mg to 3000 mg in divided doses bid or TID; start at 250 mg daily for seven days and titrate up to 2000 mg daily
- Use **nonflush niacin** or give with ASA 325 mg 30 minutes before medication to prevent flushing
- <u>**Caution diabetics!**</u>
- Monitor LFTs, glucose, and uric acid (can cause gout) at baseline and six to eight weeks after patient is on desired dose, then annually
- <u>No not give with statins</u> for increased risk of myopathy and rhabdomyolysis

## Hypertension

- See JNC eight guidelines for management
- Know the secondary causes for HTN such as renal artery stenosis, CKD, adrenal tumors, and Cushing's disease
- **Keep in mind that diuretics such as hydrochlorothiazide put patients at risk for hyperglycemia, gout, and hypercalcemia**

## Idiopathic Systolic Hypertension

- Can be caused by stiff arteries, an overactive thyroid, or diabetes; usually occurs in someone over the age of 60
- Goal systolic BP for patients over 60 is less than 150 systolic

**Management**: First-line treatment is a <u>calcium channel blocker</u>!

## JNC Eight Guidelines Pearls

- Patients < 60 years old BP goal <140/90
- Patients > 60 years old BP goal <150/90
- **Patients with diabetes, CKD goal < 140/90 and start an ACEI or ARB for HTN management**
- Nonblack patients start thiazide, ACEI, ARB, or CCB alone or in combo for BP
- Black patients start thiazide or CCB alone or in combo
- Consider lifestyle changes for all patients

## PAD/PVD

- PAD is the most common cause of atherosclerosis
- Patient may present with intermittent claudication and pain with activity that goes away with rest
- PVD: Patients legs look edematous and dark; be sure to recommend compression stockings and leg elevation for venous return

**What to know for the exam**: Lifestyle changes and daily ambulation exercise should be your recommendation. Revascularization is recommended if these therapies are not successful. Smoking cessation is crucial!

**First test to order ankle brachial index (ABI). < 0.9 is positive**

## Pulsus Paradoxus

- Occurs in patients with pericardial disease; this occurs because there is a competition between the right and left sides of the heart for space, which causes a decrease in the systolic blood pressure by < 10mm Hg during inspiration

## Prinzmetal's Angina

- Also known as variant angina; angina (chest pain) that occurs at rest, which is caused by vasospasm in the smooth muscle tissue in the vessel walls instead of being caused by atherosclerosis
- This occurs in younger patients with lower cardiac risk; exam findings are usually normal
- Symptoms occur at rest and not on exertion; may also occur in clusters
- Symptoms can occur with stress, cold exposure, cocaine abuse, and smoking
- Exercise stress test will be negative
- Typically diagnosed when other causes of chest pain have been ruled out
- Treated with calcium antagonist and nitrates

# STEMI/Non-STEMI

- **You must know** what a STEMI and a non-STEMI look like on an EKG strip
- Need to know s/s of MI such as chest pain, dyspnea, pallor, diaphoresis, n/v and that patient will have an <u>Elevated Troponin I</u>
- STEMIs present with ST elevation and carries a great risk of death and disability
- Non-STEMIs occur when the artery is partially blocked, and there is a major reduction in blood flow to the heart; ST depression is seen with non-STEMIs

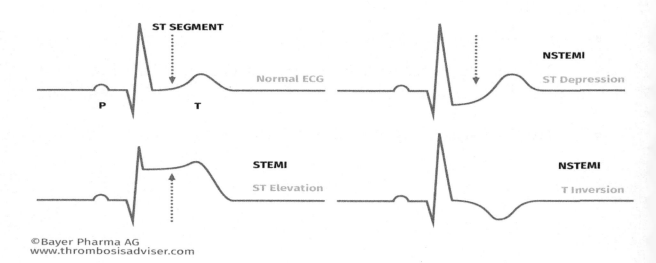

©Bayer Pharma AG
www.thrombosisadviser.com

# Dermatology

## Acne

- Most common in adolescents
- Occurs more frequent in females, patients with PCOS, obesity, and IR
- **Dietary consumption of chocolate does NOT cause acne**
- Lesions range from white and blackheads, papules to cysts
- Treated with topical retinoids and topical antibiotics; severe cases may require oral antibiotics or oral retinoid

**What to know for the exam:** Causes and treatment

## Actinic Keratosis

- Can appear as one or more lesions that occur on the face, lips, hands, forearms, and other skin-exposed regions
- **Presents as scaly macule or papule lesions that are irregularly shaped and 1 to 5 mm in diameter;** may be red or yellow in color
- Usually occurs in middle-aged or older light complicated men
- Has the potential to progress to invasive squamous cell carcinoma (SCC)

**What to know for the exam**: Remember where these lesions occur and how they present to be able to tell this from other lesions like SCC or BCC.

## Animal bites

- Typically occur on face, hands, or arms; treat animal scratches the same as animal bites
- Assess for tetanus and rabies immunization needs
- Obtain wound cultures and x-rays as needed
- Clean the wound with soap and water and then irrigate it by using an 18-gauge needle and large syringe filled with normal saline
- In general, you would not close an infected wound, especially if it occurred more than 24 hours prior to the patient visit
- Typically managed with Augmentin 500 mg/125 mg TID for five to seven days

## Basal Cell Carcinoma

- Appears as a pearly white papule nodule. patient will have increased sun exposure, so expect this in mailmen and surfers; may be described as a waxy pearly gray lesion
- Usually uncomplicated if treated properly

**What to know for the exam:** Presentation and patient scenario. This is the MOST common skin malignancy in the United States.

## Cellulitis

- Infectious skin disorder that presents with erythema, warmth, pain, and usually in the patient's extremities
- Usually caused by streptococci and staphylococcus aureus
- Mainstay of treatment is oral antibiotics depending on infectious organism

## Erysipelas

- Skin infection that presents with shiny, raised, indurated, and painful lesions <u>with distinct margins</u>; it is clinically diagnosed
- Usually caused by group A or B hemolytic streptococci
- Occurs on the face and legs
- Treated with PCN for presentation on the lower extremities and Vancomycin for facial presentations or if MRSA is suspected

**What to know for the exam:** Need to be able to differentiate between cellulitis and Erysipelas. *<u>Cellulitis is poorly demarcated and erysipelas is not.</u>*

## Fifth disease (Erythema infectiosum)

- "Slapped cheek" appearance is the most common presentation; patient may also have an erythematous rash on their extremities with mild viral symptoms
- This viral illness is caused by **parvovirus B 19**
- Typically, does not require treatment besides reassurance and symptom management
- **If this occurs in pregnancy, it could lead to fetal anemia, hydrops fetalis, or intrauterine death**

**What to know for the exam:** What can happen in pregnancy? Causative agent and presentation. Once <u>*rash appears, child is no longer contagious*</u> and may attend school. If you have an adult that presents with suspected fifth disease, draw B19 antibodies.

## Folliculitis

- Inflammation of the hair follicle; umbilicated flesh-toned papules
- Caused by bacteria, fungus, viruses and parasites; usually caused by staph aureus
- Treated with oral antibiotics such as cephalexin 250 to 500 mg QID for 10 days; also topical antibiotics or antifungals are used

**What to know for the exam:** Presentation and treatment.

## Subungual Hematoma

- Collection of blood under a toenail or fingernail caused by blunt trauma
- If the patient's nail edge is intact, and he or she is having pain, you can perform drainage to alleviate their symptoms
- Acrylic nails are a contraindication to drainage
- Drainage does not require anesthesia, but you can perform a nerve block if needed
- Use an 18-gauge needle, electrocautery device, or a paper clip and sterilized flame; clean area with povidone-iodine solution and cover with bacitracin and gauze
- Make a hole at the base of the nail or in the center of the hematoma that is large enough for the hematoma to drain

## Hand, Foot, and Mouth Disease

- Common childhood virus which is usually caused by coxasackievirus A16
- Typically resolves on its own with supportive therapy after 10 to 14 days
- Rash appears on cheeks, palms, and soles of feet
  Patient will have sores in mouth and low-grade fever
  **What to know for the exam:** Supportive management. Do not give ASA.

## Impetigo

- Bacterial skin infection commonly occurs in children and is contagious
- Typically caused by staph or strep infections

- Child will have crusting around vesicles or bullae that is itchy and painful usually found around nose or mouth
- Typically treated with topical antibiotics (mupirocin topical) and good skin hygiene

## Kawasaki Disease

- Almost always affects young children; peaks in the toddler age group
- Etiology is unknown; child typically has a high fever that has lasted longer than five days
- Child presents with polymorphic rash, conjunctivitis or injected eyes, <u>strawberry tongue</u>, and swelling and erythema in hands and feet
- The one childhood illness treated with ASA and/or IV immunoglobulin

**What to know for the exam:** Presentation!

## Lyme Disease

- Caused by a spirochete of genus Borrelia; found on animals and humans
- Initial presentation is **erythema migrans rash; this is also the most common presentation occurring in 50%–90% of patients.**
Patient may also present with fever, headache, myalgias, fatigue, and arthralgia
Flu-like symptoms presentation
Treated with <u>doxycycline 100 mg bid for 10–21 days</u>; usually treated for 14 days

**What to know for the exam:** Skin lesion present with central clearing. How to treat. Know bull's-eye rash.

## Melanoma

- Appears in a variation of colors such as brown, black, blue, gray, or red; SK is usually only brown or black
- Third most common skin cancer
- Presents with the ABCDE signs in a patient with lots of sun exposure
- Usually occurs in a person with light-colored skin

## Molluscum Contagiosum

- Transferred from skin to skin contact in kids; in adults, this is sexually transmitted; commonly found on the face, groin, and abdomen
- Patient presents with umbilicated, smooth papules that are pearl-like in nature and lesions are itchy
- Clinically diagnosed; heals on its own after weeks

**What to know for the exam:** Do nothing. Heals on its own.

## Morbilliform Rash

- Drug eruption rash
- Symmetric eruption of small papules or red macules that occur about one week after starting a new drug
- Lesions are fixed and **do not itch**
- Prevalent in children

**What to know for the exam:** Usually occurs after a person with mono receives amoxicillin or ampicillin.

## Pityriasis Rosea

- Cause is unknown
- Typically occurs in people age 10–35 years old
- Single large lesion that resemble a Christmas tree and is **known as a Herald patch**; rash is itchy and located on trunk or upper extremities
- Can last up to five months
- Treated with topical steroids, UV light treatments, and/or oral antihistamines

## Psoriasis

- Chronic inflammatory skin disease
- Patient presents with circumscribed scaly red or gray plaques or papules
- May be described as silvery scales
- Usually on knees, elbows, scalp, and extremities
- Treated with topical corticosteroids, phototherapy, methotrexate, and biologic agents

**What to know for the exam:** Presentation.

## Rocky Mountain Spotted Fever (RMSF)

- Transmitted through dog or wood tick bites; happens in spring and summer time
- Patient presents with common cold symptoms which makes it hard to diagnose patient may have fever, headache, myalgias, rash, vomiting, and a h/o a tick bite
- Treated with Doxycyclinel; effective if used in the first five days
- Triad of symptoms include fever, rash, and tick exposure

**What to know for the exam**: Treatment and s/s. Treatment is almost always Doxycycline in all age groups.

## Rosacea

- Chronic skin disorder that presents with redness, flushing, which may be described as blushing, rough skin, telangiectasia, and general inflammation that resembles acne; typically appears on the central face; especially the cheeks, chin, nose, and forehead

- Patient is usually light-skinned or older adult
- Treatment is topical metronidazole gel

**What to know for the exam:** Treatment and presentation.

## Roseola

- Common febrile illness that occurs in infants and early childhood. Caused by human herpesvirus (HHV) 6B or HHV-7.
- Patient presents with a high fever for three to five days, which is followed by a rash with discrete pinkish reddish rash that begins on the neck and trunk and spreads down to the extremities
- Rash does NOT itch
- This is self-limiting but is associated with febrile seizures

**What to know for the exam:** Rash appears AFTER days of having a fever.

## Rubella (Three-Day German Measles)

- Mild, self-limiting, viral infection caused by the rubella virus
- Patient presents with mild fever, generalized rash, lymphadenopathy, arthralgias and conjunctivitis
- If this occurs in pregnancy, it can lead to spontaneous abortion, fetal death, or a variety of anatomic and laboratory anomalies

**What to know for the exam:** What happens in pregnancy and patient presentation.

## Rubeola

- Highly infectious measles virus that has an incubation period of 10 days
- Patient presents with maculopapular rash, cough, coryza, conjunctivitis and pathognomonic enanthem, or **Koplik spots**
- Prevent by MMR

**What to know for the exam:** Koplik spots, which are red spots with a blue to white central dot found on the buccal mucosa. Remember Rube**o**la has an "O" in it for K**o**plik sp**o**ts.

## Scabies

- Transmitted from skin-to-skin contact in people living in overcrowded areas; think homeless shelters or jails
- Presentation includes intense pruritus, which may be worse at night, positive burrows, and papules on face, neck, palms, and soles of the feet
- Can occur in anyone but usually infants, children, and elderly
- Treated with permethrin or Ivermectin as a first choice

**What to know for the exam:** Treatment and presentation.

## Scarlet Fever

- Sandpaper rash seen in a child who has strep throat
- Treated with PCN

## Seborrheic Dermatitis (SD)

- Typically presents as scaling, flaking, and erythema that occurs on the scalp, nose, central face, or anterior chest

- In infants, this is called "cradle cap"; occurs in immunocompromised patients and infants < 3 months old
- Use emollients (olive oil or coconut oil) or topical steroids; if SD is limited to the scalp use topical shampoos (pyrithione zinc topical, coal tar topical, salicylic acid topical, selenium sulfide topical, etc.)

## Seborrheic Keratosis (SK)

- Brown to black waxy or scaly wart like lesions; common and usually occur in people over 50 years old
- Appears to be "stuck on" plaques or papules and may look like warts
- Benign in nature and do not usually require treatment; lesions may itch
- Rule out malignant melanoma.

**What to know for the exam:** Wart-like appearance.

## Shingles (Herpes Zoster)

- Caused by varicella zoster virus
- Patient presents with nerve-like pain or burning sensation, which is followed by a vesicular rash in the dermatome; rash will be itchy and can crust over; clinically diagnosed
- **Herpetic neuralgia can last for months after herpes zoster outbreaks and is managed as above and with acetaminophen, NSAIDS, and topical capsaicin**
- Treated with acyclovir to decrease viral replication and pain medication

**What to know for the exam**: Refer any eye involvement to the ophthalmologist urgently. Know that pain can persist after the rash is gone and the rash eruption itself is painful. Know herpetic neuralgia.

## Squamous Cell Carcinoma (SCC)

- Usually presents in a patient who has significant sun exposure; may present after a sun burn; usually the patient is older as well
- Lesion may crust or bleed and have evidence of sun damage to the skin; patient has erythematous papules or plaques on sun exposed skin areas
- May present on the patients finger or nose
  Patient may have dome-shaped nodules

## Steven–Johnson Syndrome

- Toxic epidermal necrolysis (TEN) that occurs usually after taking anticonvulsants, antibiotics, and NSAIDS.
- Patient may present with skin sloughing off (Nikolsky sign) when pressure is applied to it.
- Abrupt patient onset of symptoms, which can range from hives, blisters, generalized rash, and may involve the oral mucosa.

## Tinea Corporis

- Superficial dermatophyte infection that is either inflammatory or non-inflammatory lesions found on the scalp, groin, palms, and soles
- Starts off as erythematous, scaly plaques that either crust, vesicle, or even bullae.
- **Treated with topical azoles and allylamines**

**What to know for the exam:** Treatment.

# ENT

## Acute Otitis Media

- Patient presents with otalgia, fever, ongoing respiratory symptoms, and may have decreased hearing
- PE reveals a bulging tympanic membrane and mobility is typically decreased
- Tympanic membrane may vary in color from white to red
- Risk increased in kids in daycare, with older siblings, younger age, and children who have been bottle-fed
- Treated with oral or rectal analgesics with a delay of antibiotic use if AOM is suspected; if confirmed use amoxicillin 80–90 mg/kg/day in divided does for 10 days with a maximum dose of 1000 mg/dose (children 2 months old and up); secondary options would be cefdiner 14 mg/kg/day for 10 days in kids >6 months of age; lastly, you can use azithromycin 10 mg/kg/day for the first day and 5 mg/kg/day for four days

**What to know for the exam**: Treatment if child has allergies to first and second options. Know that strep pneumonia is the most common cause of bacterial AOM.

# Allergic Rhinitis

- Patient presents with nasal congestion, sneezing and itching nose, palate, and eyes
- Increased risk in patients with a f/h of atopy and kids
- Use topical nasal spray or antihistamines orally plus avoidance of allergen

## Air Conduction (Rinne & Webber Test)

### Causes of sensorineural loss

- Presbycusis
- Aminoglycosides
- Meningitis
- Paget's disease
- **Acoustic neuroma**

### Causes of conductive loss

- Wax
- Chronic serous otitis media
- Acute otitis media
- Otosclerosis

## Rinne Test

- Place tuning fork on mastoid process and then in front of the external canal; assess patient to see which one is louder; air conduction should be better than bone conduction; always perform the Weber test as well to r/o sensorineural hearing loss
- **AC>BC = Positive Rinne, which is normal and expected**
- BC>AC = Negative Rinne, which is seen in conductive hearing loss

## Weber Test

- Place tuning fork on the center of the forehead; sound should be heard in the middle of the patient's head.
- The sound is even in both ears in a normal Weber test.
- <u>In conductive hearing loss, the sound is heard loudest in the affected</u> ear or the more severe ear if both ears are affected

**What to know for the exam:** Conductive hearing loss Rinne is negative, and Weber localizes to affected ear. Weber test lateralization to the better ear in Meniere's disease. Cranial nerve eight test for hearing. In sensorineural hearing loss, the healthy or normal ear will have lateralization to the good ear, and the weaker ear will have sensorineural hearing loss with the Weber test. Know causes of both conductive and sensorineural hearing loss.

## Meniere's Disease

- Sudden onset of vertigo with hearing loss and tinnitus
- Patient's ear feels full
- Clinically diagnosed after other causes are ruled out
- Use pure-tone air and bone conduction with masking to help diagnose
- Use a low salt diet; less than 1500 mg to 2000 mg daily
- Diuretics such as triamterene/hydrochlorothiazide or acetazolamide

**What to know for the exam:** Weber test lateralization to the good ear, and Rinne test AC>BC is normal. Know that you can see horizontal nystagmus with Meniere's disease in acute attacks.

## Miscellaneous

- Think of cocaine abuse in adolescents with nasal turbinates that are gone
- Know nasal polyps' presentation and causes

## Mononucleosis

- Viral syndrome characterized by fever, sore throat, cervical lymphadenopathy and lymphocytosis
- **Positive heterophile** Antibody test and positive antibodies for EBV are diagnostic
- Treatment is symptom management and rest
- Perform an U/S of the spleen before patient can return to sports

**What to know for the exam:** Never treat with amoxicillin. Know the rash can occur. Know to keep patient out of contact sports until u/s confirms there is no spleen enlargement. Typically, athletes refrain from sports for three to four weeks after symptoms have resolved and their u/s of the spleen is negative.

## Otitis Externa

- **Targus pain** and tenderness
- Ear canal swelling and erythema
- Decreased hearing
- Seen frequently in swimmers and diabetics
- Use Cipro otic drops or ofloxacin otic drops
- Use ibuprofen and/or acetaminophen for pain

## Otitis Media with Effusion

- Collection of fluid behind the eardrum in the middle ear
- **Occurs WITHOUT an ear infection or after an ear infection**

- After an ear infection, remember that fluid can stay in the middle ear for a few days to weeks
- Also caused by allergies, respiratory infections, and respiratory irritants
- Typically affects children
- Patient will be asymptomatic or have mild symptoms and c/o of hearing muffled sounds
- On exam, you will see a dull TM with fluid behind the eardrum. The TM will not move with an acoustic otoscope
- **Requires no management; resolves on its own after three months**

**What to know for the exam:** Presentation and management

## Peritonsillar Abscess

- Affects children and adults
- Patient presents with a progressively worse pharyngitis, which hurts more on one side then the other when they swallow. patient may have a hot potato voice, neck pain, headaches and fever
- Usually occurs as a result of **undertreated tonsillitis**; usually caused by strep, staph, and haemophilus infections
- Treated by surgical I & D and antibiotics

## Pharyngitis

- Can be caused by viruses and bacteria
- Bacterial infections more prevalent in the winter and spring; bacterial presents with sore throat that happens **without** nasal congestion and discharge
- Goal with group A strep is to prevent rheumatic fever, transmission, and decrease the length of symptoms

- Patient presents with sore throat, cervical lymphadenopathy and exudates.
- Only use prophylactic antibiotics to prevent GAS in patients with a known history of GAS.
- First test to order is a rapid strep
- Treated with PCN

**What to know for the exam:** Do not prophylactically treat a negative rapid strep test. Treatment details. On exam, patient may have a lack of a cough. If a patient with viral pharyngitis returns with worse symptoms you would suspect strep.

## Presbycusis

- Most common type of sensorineural hearing loss that occurs from aging
- Decreased ability to hear higher-pitched frequencies
- Weber test will lateralize to the good ear
- Rinne test will be normal or AC>BC

## Sinusitis

- Acute sinusitis last >10 days but < 4 weeks and is usually caused by bacteria if it lasts that long
- Majority of cases are viral
- <u>Only use antibiotics in patients with severe disease or who are immunocompromised</u>
- Patient presents with purulent nasal drainage, facial pain and pressure, cough, sore throat and myalgias
- Treated with PCN if presentation is bacterial
- Refer patients out that present with sinusitis with periorbital cellulitis for increased intracranial pressure

# Endocrinology

## Addison Disease

- Primary adrenal insufficiency
- Patient presents with fatigue, weakness, weight loss, and **salt craving**
- Patient will be hypotensive
- Check morning cortisol test which will be low
- Treated with dexamethasone sodium phosphate 4mg IV daily for one to three days followed by hydrocortisone sodium succinate 50 to 100 mg TID or QID for one to three days if your patient is in adrenal crisis; these patients also receive 2–4 liters of IV fluid to correct underlying dehydration if needed
- Patients who are not in crisis are treated with cortisone 10 mg to 37.5 mg daily in divided doses at 8 a.m. and noon; last dose is given no later than 4 p.m.

## Cushing Syndrome

- Pathologic hypercortisolism
- Patient presents with central obesity, moon face, thin skin, muscle weakness, irregular menstrual cycles, and striae
- Key diagnostic test would be late night **cortisol** elevation and elevated 24-hour urinary cortisol level
- Refer this patient out

**What to know for the exam:** Presentation and diagnostic testing.

## Dawn Phenomenon

- Natural release of blood sugar that occurs in the early morning hours between 2a.m. and 8a.m. in order to allow your body to wake up. Typically affects diabetes and controlled by insulin.
- Can be the cause of elevated Fasting blood sugars in diabetics as their bodies are not producing enough insulin on its own.

## Diabetes

- Type 1 diabetes is managed with insulin alone
- Type 2 diabetes most prevalent type
- Patient may be asymptomatic or present with polyuria, polydipsia, polyphagia, fatigue, visual changes, paresthesia, and weight loss
- Confirmed by A1C equal to or > 6.5; note, A1C can be falsely elevated in pregnancy and anemia; a random glucose of > 200 is also confirmatory; fasting blood sugar > 125 x2 is diagnostic as well
- In pregnancy, a two-hour post glucose challenge test with 75 grams of glucose > 200 is diagnostic; this is managed with diet and basal insulin
- Type 2 diabetics with blood sugars > 300 or A1C > 10 should be started on basal insulin plus you need to reduce their cardiovascular disease risk; may add metformin as well
- First oral drug of choice is Metformin
- Note that metformin can reduce an A1C by 1% to 2%; start low and titrate your way up to 2000mg daily over a two-week period of time to avoid GI upset; if GFR is < 45 to begin with do not start metformin; **Stop metformin before surgery or if your patient is receiving**

**contrast and restart it once normal renal function is documented, as it can cause lactic acidosis, which could lead to death**
- Remember the half-life, peak, and duration of all forms of insulin
- Sulfonylureas such as glipizide, glyburide and glimepiride **work by making the pancreatic islet beta cell produce insulin**; this can cause hypoglycemia. Do not give with insulin!
- Once type-2 DM is diagnosed you order an urine microalbumin to assess kidney issues and monitor this yearly

## Hypoparthyroidism

- Occurs when there is a deficiency in a patient's parathyroid hormone (PTH) production; this causes low calcium and low albumin levels with elevated serum phosphate levels
- Can be genetic or occur post parathyroidectomy
- Patient presentations vary from asymptomatic to muscle twitches/spams, memory issues, paresthesia, and slow thinking
- **Assess for a Chvostek sign and Trousseau sign**
- **Check serum calcium and albumin, PTH**, magnesium, vitamin D, phosphorus and kidney function
- **Refer for treatment**

  **What to know for the exam**: Labs to check. PTH will be low or normal. Calcium will be low.

## Hypothyroidism

- Occurs when there is an under production of thyroid hormones
- Occurs more frequently in women and patients > 50 years old
- Patient my present with fatigue, dry skin hair and nails, depression, cold intolerance, weight gain, and lethargy
- **First test to order is a TSH which will be elevated**

- Add a T4 if your patients TSH is elevated; if it is normal then your patient has <u>subclinical hypothyroidism</u>, which you would not treat until their TSH is >10
- If the patient's T4 is low and his or her TSH is high then the patient has hypothyroidism
- You can also check a lipid panel, thyroid antibodies and fasting glucose levels
- <u>Repeat Thyroid labs in 6 to 8 week after staring medication.</u>
- Healthy patients can be started on levothyroxine 1.6 mcg per kg, which can be titrated by 12.5 mcg to 25 mcg until TSH is normal

**What to know for the exam:** Check a TSH first. Know subclinical hypothyroidism. Know when to adjust thyroid dose based on lab results.

## Hyperthyroidism (Graves' Disease)

- Autoimmune disorder where the patient's antibodies cause the patient to have an overactive thyroid
- Patient presents with unintentional weight loss, tachycardia or heart palpitations, tremor, increased sweating, heat intolerance, goiter, and upper eyelid retraction
- **TSH is the first test ordered and will be low; free T4 and T3 will be elevated**
- Thyroid storm is treated with high dose anti-thyroid meds with beta blockers, which inhibit the conversion of T4 to T3 and slows down the patient's heart; patients are also treated with radioactive iodine

- Nonemergent Graves' disease can be managed with methimazole 10 to 30 mg daily in one to three divided doses; Propylthiouracil is a secondary choice
- These patients are typically managed by endocrinology

## Hyperparathyroidism

- Can be primary or secondary; over-production of PTH hormone, which interferes with the body's ability to metabolize calcium
- Patient may present with anxiety, bone pain, insomnia, fatigue, depression, muscle pain, paresthesias, and memory issues
- **First test ordered PTH intact and serum calcium, which will both be elevated**
- Managed with parathyroidectomy and calcium and creatinine monitoring annually with bone density scans every two years for those who refuse surgery

## Metabolic Syndrome

- Includes insulin resistance, abdominal obesity, high triglycerides, HTN, and low HDLs
- Patients with PCOS, tobacco abuse, sedentary lifestyles, diets high in saturated fat, and carbohydrates are most at risk
- Check fasting glucose and fasting lipids; obtain BP, BMI and waist-to-hip ratio
- **Managed with lifestyle changes and weight loss**

## Somogyi Effect

- When a patient's blood sugar drops too low during the morning hours, the body release glucose to correct their hypoglycemia and his or her a.m. fasting sugar ends up being higher than expected; for example, if a patient took insulin at night and did not have a meal with it and they became hypoglycemic during their sleep, this could help the patient to maintain their blood sugar. (Rebound hyperglycemia)
- To differentiate between Dawn Phenomenon and Somogyi effect, you would need glucose readings at bedtime and in the very early morning hours (2 a.m. and 3 a.m.); if the patient's blood sugar is low at 2 a.m. and 3 a.m. and high at 8 a.m., then you would suspect a Somogyi effect; if the patient's blood sugar is normal at 2 a.m. and 3 a.m. and high at 8 a.m., suspect a Dawn phenomenon.

# Eye Disorders

## Blepharitis

- Inflammation of the eyelids
- Patient presents with a feeling of a foreign body sensation, burning and itching of the eye lids; there is usually crusting around the eyelashes
- Treatment consists of eyelid hygiene by applying baby shampoo
- More severe cases are treated with topical antibiotics or topical corticosteroid therapy

**What to know for the exam:** Use baby shampoo to treat

## Cataracts

- Cloudy opacity of the crystalline lens that usually occurs from normal aging
- Increased risk in those > 65 years old, **smokers, diabetics,** and patients with a h/o long-term steroid use
- Patient presents with decreased visual acuity, cloudy vision and defects in his or her red reflex
- Diagnosed with a dilated fundus exam (should be normal), glare vision test (should be significantly abnormal) and a slit lamp exam
- Refer

## Conjunctivitis

- Can be allergic, bacterial, or viral
- Allergic conjunctivitis presents with itching as the predominant symptom; use artificial tears and cold compresses to treat mild cases; use mast cell stabilizers and antihistamines for moderate to severe cases

- Viral conjunctivitis presents with watery discharge as the main symptom; use artificial tears and topical antihistamines to treat; also treated with topical corticosteroids
- Bacterial conjunctivitis has purulent discharge as the main symptom; use broad spectrum antibiotics topically to treat this
- Have contact lens wearers dispose of their contacts and use a topical fluoroquinolone such as Cipro drops

**What to know for the exam:** Know mast cell stabilizers by name such as Almast, Alomide, Opticrom and Cromolyn Sodium. Know presentation and treatment for all three.

## Corneal Abrasion

- **First thing that should be assessed is visual acuity**
- Diagnosed with fluorescein staining
- Caused by trauma, foreign bodies, and contacts lens or can occur spontaneously
- Patient presents with a sudden onset of pain and patient will have a foreign body sensation
- Usually resolved within one to two days after starting topical antibiotics
- Patients wearing contacts need to follow up with ophthalmologist in one to two days
- Know patient education for corneal abrasions such as protective eye wear, removal of contact lenses and regular eye exams

**What to know for the exam:** How to treat and know that you must assess visual acuity

## Dacrocystitis

- Infection or inflammation of the nasolacrimal sac
- Nasolacrimal duct may be blocked as well

- Can be acute or chronic
- Patient presents with excessive tearing, purulent discharge that may be yellow and crust
- Patient's eye will be watery, painful and present with redness and swelling.
- Usually occurs on the left side
- Caused by staph aureus most commonly
- In infants, have parents massage the tear ducts and use warm compresses
- At times, oral or topical antibiotics are required
- In adults, surgery may be required

**What to know for the exam:** patient may present with copious discharge at their inner canthus of the eye.

## Glaucoma

- Open-angle glaucoma typically found on routine screening
- Second leading cause of blindness in the word
- Can lead to peripheral and central vision loss if untreated
- Patient can present with peripheral vision loss but are usually asymptomatic
- **Diagnosed with tonometry** and direct ophthalmoscopy; refer to ophthalmology

- Ratio over 0.6 is suspicious for glaucoma
- Closed angle occurs when there is sudden blockage of the aqueous humor which causes increased IOP; patient presents with blurred vision, painful red eye with headache with nausea and vomiting. **Medical emergency! Send to the ER!**

**What to know for the exam:** Know to refer closed angle glaucoma to the ER and open angle to the ophthalmologist. Remember that anti-cholinergic drugs such as Spiriva (tiotropium bromide) can cause closed angle glaucoma. Use Tonometry to diagnose.

## Hirschberg Test

- Screening test that shows if a person has strabismus
- Shine a light in the patient's eyes to see where the light reflects off the cornea
- Compare the light reflexes in both eyes to determine exotropia or esotropia

## Hordeolum

- Also known as a sty
- Acute inflamed abscess on the upper or lower eye lid; usually caused by staph infections
- Tender with palpation
- Resolves with warm compress and topical antibiotics
- Can be confused with a chalazion, which is usually caused by a foreign body reaction and not tender on palpation

## Macular Degeneration

- Patient presents with sudden onset of blurring or distorted vision.
- Common in elderly
- **Loss of central vision**
- Use Amsler grid to diagnose or optical coherence tomography

**What to know for the exam**: Patient loses central vision. Use Amsler grid to diagnose.

# Miscellaneous EYE info to know

- **Cranial nerves 3, 4, and 6 are responsible for extraocular movements**
- Horizontal nystagmus that is seen for a few seconds is considered a normal finding
- Papilledema presents as blurring of the margins seen on funduscopic exam
- Know funduscopic exam findings that is normal and abnormal

## Papilledema

- Caused from increased pressure around the brain that puts pressure on the optic nerve thus causing the eyes to swell
- Patient presents with visual disturbance, headache and vomiting; may c/o blurred vision on and off, double vision, and flickering vision
- Caused by brain tumors, head trauma, bleeding in the brain, intracranial hypertension, and uncontrolled life-threatening HTN
- Treat the underlying cause

## Strabismus

- Visual axes of the eyes are misaligned
- Causes diplopia, amblyopia, and visual confusion
- **Assessed using the cover and uncover test**
- Treated by using glasses, vision therapy, eye patches and surgery in addition to correcting the underlying amblyopia and diplopia.

## Retinal Detachment

- Patient presents with a sudden loss of vision in one eye that he or she may describe as feeling blind or feeling like **a curtain has been pulled down over his or her eye**
- Patient may have floaters, flashes of lights, low central vision, and low peripheral vision
- Send to the ER

## Uveitis

- Inflammation of the iris and ciliary body
- Can lead to blindness so must be referred to ophthalmologist
- Diagnosed clinically
- Patient presents with a red eye without discharge. Patient will have pain, photophobia, blurred vision and tearing; patient may have floaters
- Assessment findings show small irregular pupils with injected conjunctiva around the corneal limbus
- Treatment includes topical steroids and treating the underlying cause

# GI/GU

## Acute Appendicitis

- Acute inflammation of the appendix which is caused by an obstruction of the lumen
- Patient presents with severe abdominal pain in the right lower quadrant, anorexia, nausea and low-grade fever
- Assess for Rovsing sign, psoas sign, and obturator sign
- **Rovsing sign:** Press down on the patient's left side of abdomen, which brings out pain on the right lower quadrant
- **Psoas sign:** Have the patient extend his or her right thigh while in the left lateral position; if that gives the patient pain in the right lower quadrant, it is a positive sign
- **Obturator sign:** Positive when pain is felt at the right lower quadrant of the patient's abdomen with internal rotation of the flexed right thigh
- Order a CT scan of the abdomen and pelvis
- Managed by appendectomy and IV antibiotics

**What to know for the exam:** Know all the signs.

## Barrett Esophagus

- Metaplasia of the intestinal epithelium which is diagnosed on biopsy
- Patients are either asymptomatic or they have GERD symptoms
- Usually seen in middle-aged White males with a h/o GERD and tobacco abuse
- Risk of cancer development depends on severity of dysplasia
- Goal is to reduce acid production but this does not reduce risk for development of cancer

- Treated with PPIs once a day or twice a day if you are treating esophagitis or twice daily dosing is required to stop GERD symptoms
- For low-grade dysplasia, radiofrequency ablation with or without endoscopy is indicated

## Campylobacter Jejuni

- Leading cause of acute diarrhea infections
- Patient presents with fever, watery diarrhea and abdominal pain; diarrhea may be bloody
- Obtain stool cultures
- Managed with supportive therapy, fluid replacement and antibiotics if symptoms persist for more than one week with high fevers
- Use macrolides, quinolones and tetracyclines; No antibiotics are indicated in mild cases
- Usually this resolves on its own after five to seven days

## Cholecystitis

- Acute inflammation of the gallbladder
- Patient presents with RUQ pain with a fever
- **Positive Murphy sign is key to diagnosing this condition**
- Palpate the patients right subcostal area and have the patient take a deep breath; if the pain and tenderness gets worse and causes respiratory arrest, this is a positive **Murphy's sign**
- You can also order a U/S
- Managed with antibiotics and cholecystectomy

**What to know for the exam:** Know the Murphy's sign and know the presentation.

## Colon Cancer

- Average risk individuals should be screened starting at age 50 and ending at age 75
- Recommendation is for a colonoscopy every 10 years, FOBT every year, CT colonography every five years or sigmoidoscopy every 10 years.
- Patient may present with pencil shaped stools **(descending colon cancer)**, blood in stool, change in bowel habit and anemia
- Surgical resection is the main treatment

## Diverticulitis

- Patient presents with <u>**left lower quadrant abdominal pain**</u>, constipation, or generalized abdominal pain
- **CT scan of the abdomen diagnostic tool of choice**
- Symptomatic uncomplicated cases are managed with two antibiotics such **as Cipro 500 mg bid and metronidazole 500 mg TID for 7 to 10 days** with a low-residue diet – and no nuts, seeds, or corn
- If case is severe (GI bleeding or not getting better after 72 hours of oral antibiotics) please refer to ER for IV antibiotics and scope

**What to know for the exam:** Imaging, presentation, and management.

## Gastric Ulcer /Peptic ulcer

- Patient presents with upper abdominal pain that may be intermittent; usually described as dull and gnawing pain
- C/o nausea or vomiting
- Pain worse with food = gastric ulcer

- Pain improved with food = peptic ulcer
- Patient may be asymptomatic with peptic ulcers
- Assess for a positive "pointing sign"
- Active bleeding ulcers or patients with red flag symptoms require a referral to the ER for endoscopy
- H. Pylori negative ulcers should be treated by discontinuing all NSAIDS unless needed for CAD; consider COX-2 inhibitor for patients with low risk for CAD
- Treat with PPI when appropriate for four weeks in patients that are negative for H. pylori and have a duodenal ulcer and for eight weeks in patients with gastric ulcers
- H. pylori requires eradication therapy; be sure red flag symptoms are absent before starting therapy; D/C NSAIDS when possible; use triple therapy with PPI such as omeprazole 20 mg BID and 2 antibiotics such as metrondidazole 500 mg QID and tetracycline 500 mg QID
- Repeat H. pylori breath test after one month of treatment

**What to know for the exam:** How to treat H. Pylori. Know the difference between duodenal and gastric ulcers.

## GERD

- Reflux of gastric contents into the esophagus
- Increased risk with obesity, NSAID use, tobacco abuse, alcohol consumption, diets high in acid, and stress
- **Standard treatment with PPIs= four to eight weeks**
- Lifestyle changes
- Suspect esophageal stricture if patient is also experiencing dysphagia

## Giardiasis

- GI infection caused by flagellated protozoan parasites
- Transferred via fecal oral route
- Patient presents with foul smelling stool, diarrhea that may be chronic, abdominal pain with bloating and belching
- Obtain a stool culture
- Treated with Tinidazole 2 g PO x 1 or metronidazole 250mg TID for five to seven days

**What to know for the exam:** Know treatment and presentation.

## Hemorrhoids

- Can be internal and external
- Patient presents with painless rectal bleeding and tender perianal mass; they may also complain of constipation and anal itching
- Treated with 25–30 gs of fiber daily and topical corticosteroids
- More severe cases are managed with rubber band ligation and surgical removal

**What to know for the exam:** Presentation and management.

## Non-Alcoholic Fatty Liver Disease (NAFLD)

- Seen in patients without alcoholism that have fatty liver infiltrate in the liver
- Can progress to cirrhosis and end stage liver disease
- Most common cause of chronic liver disease in the Western world
- Patients typically have obesity and metabolic syndrome
- Lifestyle changes first line therapy

## Proteinuria

- Commonly occurs as kidney function decreases to a GFR of < 90
- More common in blacks than whites
- Urine dipstick can be falsely negative
- Test patients with chronic kidney disease, HTN, DM and reduced kidney function on a yearly basis
- Screen type 1 diabetics annually after five years of onset of the disease
- Persistent proteinuria is suspected when a patient is positive for protein on two urine samples one to two weeks apart
- Direct measurement with a **24-hour urine protein-to-creatine ratio** is the next lab to test for patients with persistent proteinuria

## Pyelonephritis

- Can be acute or chronic inflammation of the kidneys
- Patient presents with a fever, nausea and vomiting, increased urination with pain and urgency, and severe flank pain
- **Patient will feel CVA tenderness on exam**
- Obtain an UA and urine C&S
- Usually caused by E coli.
- Managed with cefixime 400 mg PO daily for two weeks, or Cipro 500 mg bid for one to two weeks, or trimethoprim/sulfamethoxaszole 160 mg/800 mg bid for two weeks

# Hematology/Oncology

## B12 Deficiency/Pernicious Anemia

- Macrocytic hyperchromic anemia
- Patient has neurological symptoms such as memory loss, paresthesias, weakness, ataxia, beefy red tongue (glossitis), and cognitive impairment
- Risk factors such as vegan and vegetarian diet, aging, h/o gastric surgery, alcoholic liver disease, and GI disorders that interfere with absorption
- Medications that cause B12 deficiency include metformin, H2 blockers, PPIs and anticonvulsants
- Order a serum B12, CBC, peripheral smear & folate level
- Antiparietal cell antibody test differentiates B 12 deficiency from pernicious anemia
- Must use IM or Subq B12 1mg for pernicious anemia & B12 deficiencies that are caused by GI disorders or GI surgeries
  **What to know for the exam:** Pernicious anemia can cause permanent cognitive impartment. Know the s/s of presentation

## Multiple Myeloma

- Cancer that affects the plasma cells and causes cancer cells to accumulate in the bone marrow
- Patient may present with **bone pain**, weight loss, poor appetite, constipation, fatigue, and frequent infections
- **Typically affects people age 60 and above**
- Obtain a CBC, which should show anemia, CMP with serum calcium (elevated) and albumin (low)

- Bone marrow biopsy
- Refer out

## Thalassemia

- Inherited microcytic anemia which is caused by mutations of the beta-globin gene; autosomal recessive trait
- Patients can range from asymptomatic to suffering from severe anemia
- **Seen in the Mediterranean, Middle East, North Africa, India, and Southeast Asia**
- Patient may present with fatigue and pallor, large head, lethargy, and small frame
- **Confirmatory test hemoglobin electrophoresis**
- Labs include CBC, peripheral smear, LFTs, and reticulocyte; you expect microcytic anemia in the presence of normal or elevated iron levels

**What to know for the exam:** Hemoglobin electrophoresis will confirm thalassemia and know the regions that are mostly commonly affected.

## Sickle Cell Anemia

- Autosomal recessive gene defect that affects hemoglobin A, where Hemoglobin S is produced instead.
- Occurs in one out of four pregnancies when both parents carry the gene.
- Tested at birth with neonatal screening.
- Commonly affects Blacks and Hispanics.

- Management focuses on symptom control and disease prevention; patients are usually managed by pain specialist for chronic pain
- In children, you want to prevent infections through proper immunizations, prophylactic antibiotics when necessary and proper hydration
- Patients can use hydroxyurea, blood transfusions, and bone marrow transplant at the hematologist discretion

# Infectious Disease/Sexually Transmitted Disease

## Anthrax

- Bacillus anthracis spores form gram positive bacillus
- Patient presents with painless, itchy papules that turn into vesicles or ulcers
- Increased risk if patient works with animals or contaminated animal products such as **farmers**
- Mail carriers were exposed when anthrax was used as a form of bioterrorism

**What to know for the exam:** Remember the people that are at risk for this such as mail carriers and farmers. Know the presentation for sure.

## Antibiotic Drug Classes

### **Antifungals**

Fluconazole

Ketoconazole

Terbinafine (Lamisil)

Nystatin

### **Antiparasitics**

Nitazoxanide

Metronidazole

Tinidazole

## Antivirals ophthalmic

Trifluridine

Ganciclovir

## First-Generation Cephalosporins

Cefadroxil

Cefazolin

Cephalexin

Cefadroxil

Cephalexin

Cefazolin

## Second-Generation Cephalosporins

Cefaclor

Cefotetan

Cefoxitin

Cefprozil

Cefuroxime axetil

Cefuroxime sodium

## Third-Generation Cephalosporins

Cefepime

Ceftolozane/tazobactam

**Fifth-Generation Cephalosporin**

Ceftaroline fosamil

**Fluoroquinolones**

Ciprofloxacin

Delafloxacin

Gemifloxacin

Levofloxacin

Ofloxacin

Macrolides

Azithromycin

Clarithromycin

Erythromycin

**Penicillins**

Amoxicillin

Ampicillin

Amoxicillin/clavulanate

Penicillin G

Penicillin V

**Tetracyclines** (Do not give to children < 8 years old)

Doxycycline

Minocycline

Vibramycin

Tetracycline

**Sulfonamides**

Sulfamethoxazole/trimethoprim

Erythromycin/sulfisoxazole

**Tuberculosis meds**

Isoniazid

Pyridoxine

Rifadin

## Bacterial Vaginosis (BV)

- Leading cause of vaginitis especially in reproductive years
- Patient presents with a fishy vaginal discharge, itching and pain with sex and urination
- **Vaginal PH is > 4.5 with BV**
- **Positive "whiff" test**
- Managed with metronidazole 500 mg bid for seven days or vaginal metronidazole 0.75% nightly for five nights
- Do not use metronidazole in the first trimester of pregnancy

## Chlamydia (STI infection)

- **Most frequently reported notifiable disease in the United States**
- Usually asymptomatic
- Women may present with yellow cervical discharge, friable cervix and abnormal vaginal bleeding.
- Men may present with mucoid penile discharge.
- **First test ordered nucleic acid amplification test (NAAT)**
- Use **azithromycin 1 g PO x 1** or doxycycline 100mg bid for seven days.
- In pregnant woman **azithromycin 1 g PO x 1** is still the primary option Alternatively, you can give amoxicillin 1 g TID for seven days as well.

## Cytomegalovirus

- Ubiquitous beta-herpes virus and is considered the fifth member of the human herpes virus family
- Patient may present with malaise, diarrhea with nausea and vomiting, fever and visual changes; patient may also be asymptomatic
- Increased risk in immunocompromised and newborns infected during pregnancy
- Obtain CBC and CMV titers
- CMV IGM positive reflects an acute infection
- CMV IgG positive reflects a past positive
- Treatment is not usually necessary unless patient is immunocompromised

## Gonorrhea

- Typically, patient presents with urethral irritation, dysuria, purulent discharge and pain with intercourse
- Culture positive
- NAAT positive for gonorrhea
- **Treated with ceftriaxone 250mg IM x 1 AND azithromycin 1 g orally x 1** Same treatment for pregnant non-complicated patients
- Add metronidazole for patients that were sexually assaulted

## Hepatitis B Virus

- **HBsAg** = Patient is in the middle of being sick; "s" in the middle means patient has an acute hepatitis infection; positive in acute and chronic infections. Shows positive after 2-10 weeks of exposure.

- **Serum anti-HBs** = Surface antibody; "s" at the end of the antibodies means the patient is immune to hepatitis B; either from having an active infection or from the immunization; either way, the patient is safe; can check anti-HBc to confirm natural infection

- **Serum anti-HBc IgM** = In this case, a positive test means the patient is miserable right this minute; the patient has a hepatitis infection that is currently infectious right now; patient would have become infected within the last six months.

- **Serum anti-HBc IgG** = In this case a positive test means the patient has an infection that is gone – either it is gone from having the immunization or an acute infection.

- **Serum HBeAg** = The hepatitis B e-antigen is positive when the virus is replicating and the person is infectious

## Herpes Simplex Virus (HSV)

- Patients usually present with genital or oral ulcer that presented with a tingling or burning feeling
- Increased risk of HSV in the immunocompromised and patients with high risk sexual behavior.
- Can obtain a viral culture, HSV PCR and HSV antibodies for HSV 1 and 2
- Treated with acyclovir, valacyclovir or famciclovir

## Herpes Zoster

- See Shingles

## HIV

- It is recommended that patients start a strong combination antiretroviral therapy (ART) regardless of CD4 count to decrease disease progression and prevent HIV transmission
- **PPD positive if equal to or > 5mm in HIV positive patients**
- If CD4 count is < 200 patient is classified as having AIDS
- **Use trimethoprim/sulfamethaoxazole 160/800mg daily as drug of choice for patients with a CD4 count <200 to prevent pneumocystis jirovecii**

## HPV (Genital Warts)

- Caused by HPV genotypes 6 and 11, although over 40 types can infect the genital area
- Must come in direct contact with the lesion whether it be clinical or subclinical in presentation

- Clinically diagnosed but you can perform a biopsy
- No cure and often reoccurs
- **Treated with podofilox topical 0.5% applied** directly to the affected area twice a day for three days then no treatment for four days; this can be repeated up to four times
- **Provider treatment consist of trichloroacetic acid topical 90%** applied directly to wart and then covered with a dressing for five to six days and repeated on a weekly basis until wart is gone; have patient wash his or her skin four hours after application.
- Routine HPV vaccines are recommended for adolescents starting at ages 9 to age 26 years old.

**What to know for the exam:** Know treatment.

## Pelvic Inflammatory Disease (PID)

- Inflammatory disorders affecting the female genital tract; when sexually transmitted, it is usually caused by N. gonorrhoeae and Chlamydia trachomatis
- Patients with a h/o STIs, younger than 24 years old, have an IUD and are sexually active with multiple sexual partners are at the greatest risk
- Patient presents with uterine tenderness, low-grade fever, and lower abdominal pain
- On exam patient will have cervical motion tenderness and adnexal tenderness
- Order STI testing and UA

- **Treated with ceftriaxone 250 mg IM x 1 and doxycycline 100mg bid for 14 days; add metronidazole for trichomonas and bacterial vaginosis**

**What to know for the exam:** Treatment.

## Pneumonia

- CAP acquired outside of the hospital
- Clinically diagnosed
- Chest x-ray shows infiltrates
- Patient presents with dyspnea, fever or chills, chest pain, cough with sputum production; usually febrile with myalgias.
- On exam you hear dullness to percussion of the affected lobe
- **Treat outpatient with macrolides** or tetracyclines first-line therapy
- Patients with comorbidities such as diabetes receive fluoroquinolones
- Repeat chest x-rays after antibiotics therapy
- Have patient contact you if his or her symptoms have not improved in 72 hours

**What to know for the exam:** What pneumonia looks like on an x-ray and treatment.

## Syphilis

- Causative agent spirochetal bacterium Treponema pallidum
- Increased risk of acquiring HIV with untreated syphilis infections
- Can cause miscarriage and still-birth
- Primary syphilis starts off as a macule that later turns into a chancre sore 10 to 90 days later

- Secondary develops four to eight weeks after primary infection; patient has rash on feet and hands that is **not itchy**
- Early latent stage occurs after secondary stage but less than one year from first exposure; patient is asymptomatic and will have positive lab results
- Late latent syphilis occurs in patients who are asymptomatic and had their first exposure more than one year ago but less than two years ago; patient is asymptomatic
- Tertiary syphilis occurs when chronic systemic infection sets in and leads to chronic end organ issues such as neurosyphilis
- Treated with IM benzathine penicillin G
- Desensitization is used for pregnant women with a PCN allergy
- **Jarish–Herxheimer reaction** can occur after antibiotic use within the first 24 hours; patient can have a fever, headache, and body aches; typically occurs in early syphilis; treated with supportive therapy, acetaminophen and NSAIDS.

**What to know for the exam:** Presentation of a chancre sore that is painless and can go away on its own without treatment. Know Jarish–Herxheimer reaction.

## Toxoplasmosis

- Protozoan parasite typically transferred to humans via infected cat feces
- Commonly seen in immunocompromised patients, such as someone with AIDS or can occur during pregnancy
- Patient may present with blurry vision, confusion, unsteady gait, and headache

- Draw anti-toxoplasma IgG and IgM titers
- Management depends on patient group

## Trichomonas

- Positive **"whiff test"** from trichomonas and bacterial vaginosis
- Female patient presents with malodorous vaginal secretions and itching with pain with urination
- Vaginal culture will be positive for trichomonas
- Treat with metronidazole 2 grams PO x 1 or tinidazole 2 grams PO x 1. Tinidazole has a longer half-life then metronidazole
- **Do not give metronidazole in the first trimester of pregnancy**

# Tuberculosis (TB)

- Patient presents with weight loss, anorexia, malaise, night sweats, fevers, and cough
- Mainly **affects the lungs** – but can affect any organ system
- Increased risk in patients with HIV, immunocompromised, exposure to TB, homelessness, and patients that are incarcerated
- Order chest x-ray, acid-fast bacilli sputum smear and sputum culture
- **TB skin test positive if equal to or > 5 mm in an HIV positive patient**
- Positive if equal to or > 10 mm in a patient with DM, tobacco abuse, alcoholism, IVDA, high-risk employee such as those working in prisons and nursing homes, and TB lab personnel.
- If > or equal to 15 with no risk factors this is a positive reading.
- Patients need to be isolated for 5 to 14 days after initial treatment and close contacts need to be evaluated and treated
- Usually treated with isoniazid daily for six to nine months or rifampin daily for four months

**What to know for the exam:** Presentation, diagnostic criteria in TB skin test and sputum collection. How to identify TB on a chest x-ray.

## Labs to Know

- **ESR (sed rate):** Elevated with inflammatory disorders; elevated in temporal arteritis, lupus, RA, and more; does not elevate with aging
- **Glucagon:** Peptide hormone produced by the pancreas; elevates glucose levels in the presence of hypoglycemia
- **IgE:** Immunoglobulin E, which is an antibody that is **elevated in patients with allergies**, asthma, and atopic dermatitis
- **Prolactin:** Check in women with amenorrhea or with galactorrhea (abnormal breast discharge); check in young men with low testosterone and gynecomastia; can also be elevated in infertility, low libido, patients with E.D and more; if serum prolactin is high, ensure patient is not on medications that can elevate prolactin levels such as GI medications and antipsychotic medications such as SSRIs; if prolactin is elevated without a cause, order an MRI of the brain to r/o a prolactinomas, which is more common in females than males; typically prolactinomas are benign and can be treated with dopamine agonists, which decrease the levels and help to shrink the tumor
- **RPR/VDRL:** Used to diagnose syphilis
- **TSH:** Test of choice for evaluating hyper and hypoactive thyroid

# Men's Health
## Benign prostatic hyperplasia (BPH)

- Patient presents with frequency, urgency, nocturia, decreased stream, straining with urination and post-void dribbling
- Prostate goes through its second growth spurt around age 50
- Check PSA and follow age-related guidelines
- On examination, a normal prostate should feel soft, smooth & symmetrical, and about the size of a walnut
- Enlarged prostates may feel boggy
- Treatment includes alpha blockers such as terazosin 1 mg Q HS, as it can cause orthostatic hypotension; increase the dose to 5 mg to 10 mg or give up to 20 mg daily max per day in a divided dose
- Note that tamsulosin (Flomax) does not cause hypotension, as it selectively relaxes the smooth muscle and improves the urine flow

**What to know for the exam:** A boggy prostate is noted during the exam. Drug choices for treatment.

## Epididymitis

- Inflammation of the epididymis
- Patient presents with pain and swelling on one side that has persisted over the course of a few days
- In men younger than 35 and sexually active this is caused by Chlamydia trachomatis or Neisseria gonorrhoeae
- Diagnosed with gram stain of urethral secretions that are collected before collecting urine specimen; you can also obtain a culture of urethral secretions
- Treated with ceftriaxone 250 mg IM x1 and doxycycline 100 mg bid for 14 days for sexually transmitted infections

- Treated with a quinolone such as levofloxacin 500 mg daily x 10 days or Ofloxacin 300 mg bid for 10 days for non-sexually transmitted injections

**What to know for the exam:** Treatment & to screen for STIs as the underlying cause.

## Miscellaneous

- SSRIs are a common cause of erectile dysfunction
- TCAs work better for depression in men

## Prostate Cancer

- Second-leading cause of cancer related deaths in the United States
- Increased incidence in Black men, patients with a first-degree relative with prostate cancer, high-fat diets and men > 50 years old
- Recent research has not linked hormone replacement with increased risk of prostate cancer; more research is needed
- Elevated PSA > 4.0 ng/ml should be referred for biopsy
- **Patient's prostate will feel firm and nodular on exam while an enlarged prostate will feel boggy**

## Testicular Cancer

- Accounts for < 1% of the cancer deaths in men
- Increased risk in patients with h/o cryptorchidism (undescended testes)
- Male patient age 20–34 presents with a **painless** testicular mass

- Order an ultrasound of the testis (very sensitive); also check a serum beta HCG; if it's > 0.7 U/L, it's positive
- Managed surgically

## Testicular Torsion

- **Urologic emergency**
- Occurs when there is twisting of the testicle on the spermatic cord, which causes ischemia
- Usually occurs in males < 25 years old and infants
- Patient presents with one-sided testicular pain, scrotal swelling, or edema and **absent cremasteric reflex**
- Send to the ER

# Mood Disorders
## Anxiety & Depression

- Ongoing anxiety and depression are both managed with SSRIs as the drug of choice (Lexapro, Paxil, Zoloft, Prozac, and Celexa)
- Can use a beta blocker such as propranolol for stage freight or speeches to help calm anxiety
- Remember ongoing caregiver stress can cause depression
- Common side effects of SSRIs include weight gain and **erectile dysfunction** and can prolong a patient's QT interval
- TCAs work better in men than in women for depression (Pamelor, amitriptyline, nortriptyline)
- **TCAs' common side-effect profile includes blurred vision, constipation, dry mouth, and urine retention**
- **Atypical antipsychotic medication such as Zyprexa, require fasting glucose and lipid panel monitoring at baseline and periodically**
- You must wean long-term benzodiazepines to discontinue
- Know the side effects of MAOIs such as Nardil, Marplan, Parnate; educate your patient that he or she must avoid alcohol, cheese, aged meats, chocolate, and other tyramine-rich foods as this can lead to hypertensive emergency when taken with an MAOI.

## Anorexia Nervosa

- Eating disorder where patient has a body image disturbance and denies his or herself food due to fear of weight gain
- Patient presents with weight loss, body image disturbance, binge, and/or purge eating disorder, misuse of laxatives and amenorrhea
- These patients are on a self-induced calorie-restricted diet
- Increase risk in adolescent females
- Draw CBC, CMP, TFT; check an UA
- Managed with balanced nutrition plan and therapy; consider fluid and electrolyte replacement in severe cases; if patient has depression you can add an SSRI such as fluoxetine or sertraline

## Bulimia Nervosa

- Eating disorder that occurs when a patient experiences episodes of binge eating followed by purging or excessive fasting/exercise
- Patient presents with recurrent episodes of binge eating with some sort of compensation to accommodate their overeating; may also have depression and self-esteem issues
- Assess for dental erosion, Russell sign (scarring over the top of hands), menstrual irregularities and etc.
- Check CBC, CMP, magnesium, serum CK and UA
- Treated with therapy, balanced diet and SSRIs or SNRIs

# Musculoskeletal Disorders

## ACL/MCL/LCL Injuries

- An injury to the MCL, ACL, or LCL usually is a sprain or tear
- Typically, a sports-related injury or an injury that occurs with bending or twisting the knee
- Patient presents with swelling, pain, and tenderness at the affected site
- Patient may have heard an audible "pop" sound
- X-rays r/o fractures and MRI's determine tears
- ACL tears feel like the knee wants to buckle or give out
- Mild injuries usually get better with supportive care and heal in one to two weeks
- Moderate injuries last four weeks or longer; May require bracing
- Severe injuries require hinged bracing for months and limited weight bearing
- Use RICE, NSAIDs, and stretching or strength exercises

## Assessment Test

**Anterior Draw Test:** Place the patient supine. Flex hips to a 45-degree angle with the knee at 90 degrees. The patient's feet should be flat on the table. You then sit on the patient's feet (yes!) and pull the tibia forward toward you. If the tibia moves more than usual, it's a positive test – not sensitive or specific, though. This test the integrity of the ACL.

**Apley Test:** Have patient lay prone and flex his or her knee to 90 degrees. Place your knee across the posterior (back) of the patient's thigh and pull patient's lower leg while externally rotating patient's foot. Pain is usually felt at the meniscus and would be considered a positive test. Positive findings usually mean there is meniscus damage.

**Ballottement test:** Have the patient lay supine with his or her leg straight. You apply pressure to the knee anteriorly and posteriorly. The patella should move about 1 mm if there is nothing wrong. More movement than 1 mm (bogginess) is considered a positive test. Positive findings show increased fluid on the suprapatellar pouch.

**Finkelstein Test:** Have the patient bend their fifth digit (thumb) of the affected hand down across their palm and then have them cover their thumb with their fingers and bend their wrist towards their little finger; pain is positive. Positive findings suspect de Quervain's tenosynovitis.

**Latchman's Test:** The most accurate test for assessing an acute ACL tear. The patient is supine, and you put your hand behind the tibia; the other hand goes on the patient's thigh. The patient's knee should be 20 to 30 degrees flexed. Place your thumb on the tibial tuberosity and pull the tibia forward or toward you. Positive test includes a soft endpoint with a 2 mm movement. Negative occurs when there is a firm endpoint.

**McMurray Test:** Place patient supine and flex his or her knee while you flex the patient's hip with one hand and place your other hand on their knee joint line. Rotate patient's foot internally and externally. Pain with rotation is a positive test. Evaluates a meniscus tear/injury.

**Ottawa Ankle Rules:** Guideline to help you determine if your patient needs an ankle x-ray after an ankle injury. If the patient has pain in the malleolar and/or at least one other assessment finding, such as bone tenderness at the tip of the lateral or medial malleolus or the patient is not able to bear weight after injury. When using these rules to assess for foot pain, the patient must have pain in his or her midfoot plus bone tenderness at the base of the fifth metatarsal or navicular or be unable to bear weight.

## Carpal Tunnel Syndrome (CTS)

- Common entrapment syndrome that causes neuropathy in the first through third digits
- Patient presents with numbness and or tingling of the first through third digits along with wrist pain
- Clinically diagnosed, but EMGs are helpful in diagnosis CTS
- **Wrist splints and NSAIDS are treatment options of choice**
- Hydrochlorothiazide and steroid injections are also used if primary choices fail

## De Quervain's Tendonitis

- Pain that affects the wrist and hand and can involve any of the tendons in either area
- Patient presents with pain in his or her dominate thumb and may state it locks or the pain may be in the wrist; gets better with rest. Commonly affects both wrist and gets worse with heavy lifting.
- Usually affects patients >50 years old
- Perform a Finkelstein's test in the office and order a high-resolution ultrasound scan outpatient
- Managed with NSAIDs/splinting, steroid injections, and lastly surgery

## Giant Cell Arteritis (Temporal Arteritis)

- Form of vasculitis that affects people age >50 and older

- Patient presents with a headache, may have partial vision loss, with pain and stiffness in the neck and shoulders
- May present with polymyalgia rheumatic symptoms
- Diagnostic criteria **temporal artery biopsy**
- Check **ESR**, CRP, CBC, and LFTs

**What to know for the exam:** Presentation and diagnostic criteria.

## Gout

- Gout can affect any joint but commonly affects the patient's great toe; occurs from hyperuricemia depositing urate crystals in the joint spaces, which causes an acute arthritis presentation.
- Occurs in older males more frequently than others
- Occurs in those whom consume a lot of meat, seafood, and alcohol
- Increase risk with the use of aspirin and diuretics
- **Patient may present with sudden onset of joint pain and stiffness with erythema and effusion; tophi are commonly seen as well**
- Order an arthrocentesis with synovial fluid analysis to confirm gout
- Uric acid levels commonly ordered in primary care; levels above 7 mg/dl in men and 6 mg/dl in women considered positive
- **Goal uric acid level is < 6 mg/dl**
- Acute gout attacks are treated with NSAIDS, corticosteroids, and colchicine
- Use the least-effective dose of colchicine and only use when patients have contraindications to NSAIDS and COX-2 inhibitors; advise patient that colchicine can cause GI upset
- Do not use allopurinol for acute gout attacks

# Osteoarthritis (OA)

- Most common form of arthritis
- Usually affects the joints in the hands, knees, hips, and lumbar spine
- Patient presents with joint pain that last about 30 minutes in the morning and gets worse with activity
- Bouchards nodes and Heberden nodes are present; **mostly affects DIP joints**
- Aerobic exercise and physical therapy are ideal nonpharmacologic treatments
- Acetaminophen and topical capsaicin or topical NSAIDS are primary pharmaceutical options

**What to know for the exam:** Affected joints and treatment.

## Osteoporosis

- **Risk factors include female gender, White race, low BMI, menopausal, vitamin D deficiency, tobacco abuse, and loss of height.**
- Prevention includes weight-bearing and aerobic exercise
- Replace calcium and vitamin D at every age
- Smoking cessation
- DXA scan should be ordered. Also order serum calcium, alk phos, thyroid function test and serum 25-hydroxy vitamin D
- T-scores <2.5 equals osteoporosis
- T-scores 1.0 to 2.4 equals osteopenia
- Managed with bisphosphonates, calcium and vitamin D supplements

**What to know for the exam:** Risk factors, prevention, and management.

## Polymyalgia Rheumatica

- Inflammatory syndrome that consist of morning pain and stiffness of the neck, shoulders, and pelvic girdle
- Can occur with giant cell arteritis, depression, and weight loss
- Affects people > 50 years old and occurs more frequently in females
- Patients typically have elevated ESR rates ranging from 30–40 and elevated CRP levels
- Managed with low dose steroids; note that NSAIDS are not recommended as a primary treatment option.

**What to know for the exam:** Check ESR and CRP and know treatment.

## RA

- Usually way more joints involved then OA and has more systemic effects
- Usually affects the MCP joints and not the DIP joints
- Longer morning stiffness – one hour or more
- Swan neck deformities
- Can co-exist with OA
- Check RF, ESR, and CRP
- Treated with Methotrexate primarily

**What to know for the exam:** Labs to check and how to differentiate this from OA.

## Shin splints

- Also referred to as medial tibial stress syndrome
- Typically occurs in runners
- Stop or decrease training or activity that causes stress
- Rest and ice
- Wrap legs before running

## Spinal stenosis

- Can be congenital or acquired from degeneration or trauma/injury
- Patient presents with c/o back pain, legs feeling heavy or pain with ambulation, numbness and tingling that radiates down the legs
- **Pain can be relieved by bending forward**
- Order an x-ray followed by an MRI for more severe cases
- Managed with surgical decompression for neuro deficits.
- Managed with gabapentin, duloxetine, other analgesics, and steroids for non-neuro involvement

# Neurology

## Assessment of the Neurological System

**Brudzinski Sign:** Have the patient flex his or her neck; if the patient involuntarily flexes knees and hips, it's a positive sign; suspect meningitis. (5% sensitive and 95% specific)

**Kernig Sign:** Have the patient lay supine and flex thigh to a 90-degree right angle; when you try to straighten the patient's knee, if he or she resists, this is a positive sign; suspect meningitis. (Seen more in children than adults)

**Romberg Test**: This test the patient's cerebellum function to maintain truncal stability with eyes closed. Essentially, you are testing their coordination and balance. Main purpose of this test is to assess a patient's proprioception (or their positioning). **Have patient put his or her feet together, arms at their sides and stand with eyes closed.** Make sure you are nearby should the patient get dizzy and want to fall.

**Mini Mental Status Test:** Assesses orientation, attention and calculation, recall, registration and language, and praxis. This assess for memory loss, cognitive impairment, and the patient's odds of having dementia.

## Bell Palsy

- Facial nerve palsy that presents on one side; rest of the exam findings are negative such as TIA or CVA symptoms
- Increased risk in the African-American population; patients who received an intranasal flu vaccine, recent URI, and pregnancy
- Can occur at any age and affects men and women equally
- Managed with corticosteroids and eye protection

**What to know for the exam:** Presentation.

## Benign Essential Tremor

- Common in early adulthood and the aging population; increased risk with family history
- Incurable
- Patient will present with symmetric involuntary tremors in the hand and forearms that goes away at rest and reappears during intentional movement
- Diagnosed clinically
- Voice, head, and jaw can be involved
- Use propranolol 10 mg to 20 mg bid with a max dose of 320 mg daily or primidone 12.5 mg to 25 mg daily with a max dose of 750 mg daily

**What to know for the exam:** Treatment and presentation.

## Dementia

- Several variations of this illness, including vascular dementia, and Alzheimer's and dementia with Lewy bodies.
- Memory loss; loss of judgment
- Patients present with forgetfulness, decreased social skills, and impaired decision-making skills
- Vascular dementia occurs in those with previous history of a CVA and only accounts for about 10% of the dementia cases
- **Dementia symptoms are gradual verses delirium symptoms**
- **With Alzheimer's, patients produce less acetylcholine than normal**

**What to know for the exam:** Use a mini mental status test to assess for probability of dementia. Think of vascular dementia in patients with an h/o CVA or DM. Know the difference between dementia and delirium.

# Headaches

**Cluster Headaches:** One of the most painful headaches. Patient presents with unilateral headache that last anywhere from 15 minutes to three hours. **Pain is typically around the orbits or temples.** Patient may also have nausea, vomiting, nasal congestion, and photophobia. Cluster headaches are managed with sumatriptan, oxygen, intranasal zolmitriptan, and more. Verapamil and lithium can be used for chronic cluster headache prophylaxis.

**Migraines** occur on one or both sides and are described as pounding pain that lasts for hours to days. Patient may have nausea, light sensitivity, and aura. Risk factors for migraines include females, menses, caffeine intake, stress, lack of sleep, and family h/o migraines. Migraines are managed with NSAIDS, antiemetics, acetaminophen, and sumatriptan if there are no contraindications.

You can **use beta blockers such as propranolol** and timolol or TCAs such as amitriptyline; sodium valporate (Depakote) and topiramate (Topamax) as prophylactic treatments.

**What to know for the exam:** Presentation of migraine headaches and prophylactic treatment options.

## Fibromyalgia

- Chronic pain syndrome
- Patients c/o pain on the front, back, right and left sides of their diaphragm, which has occurred for a minimum of three months. Patient will also have at least 11 out of 18 tender points
- Patient can present with a number of issues such as insomnia or hypersomnia, fatigue despite rest, issues with mood, numbness/tingling sensations, unexplained pain and wide spread tenderness on examination
- Clinically diagnosed
- Check ESR, Sed rate, ANA, RF, and CCP to rule out other causes of chronic pain
- Usually managed with TCAs, SNRIs, muscle relaxers, and others

**What to know for the exam:** How to diagnose.

## Meningitis (Bacterial)

- Caused by streptococcus pneumoniae, H. influenza and Neisseria meningitis
- Typically affects the really young and the older population
- Patient can present with a **severe headache, neck stiffness, fever, confusion,** and more
- **Nuchal rigidity found on exam**
- Positive Kernig sign or Brudzinski sign
- Diagnosed with CSF showing elevated protein, low glucose and a positive gram stain and culture
- Managed with age appropriate IV antibiotics

**What to know for the exam**: Presentation, special test, and exam findings.

## Multiple Sclerosis

- <u>**Inflammatory demyelinating disease**</u> that affects two of the following areas: brain, spinal cord, and optic nerves
- Occurs more frequently in females aged 20–40 years old
- Patient may present with fatigue, polyuria, spastic muscle tone, balance and coordination issues, and visual disturbance in one eye
- Order an MRI of the brain and cervical spine to assess for demyelination.
- **Managed with immunomodulators such as interferon, antispasmodic medications, and regular exercise with sleep hygiene**
- Methylprednisolone is used for acute flares

## Myasthenia Gravis

- Auto-immune disorder that affects the connection between the nervous and musculoskeletal system
- Cause is unknown but could stem from viral and bacterial infections
- Affects women more than men
- **Presentation includes muscle weakness in the eyes, face, neck and limbs; patient may have ptosis, visual changes, difficulty swallowing and breathing; Symptoms spread from the patients face-down**
- Check a serum acetylcholine receptor antibody analysis
- Mild to moderate cases are managed with **pyridostigmine (anticholinergic) and immunosuppressants**

**What to know for the exam:** Know the patient presentation and treatment.

## Trigeminal Neuralgia

- Facial pain syndrome that affect the trigeminal nerve region
- Patients c/o sharp shooting or stabbing pain that last about two minutes at a time
- Patient may complain that facial touch or cold air makes symptoms worse
- Clinically diagnosed, as patient will not have any other neurological symptoms
- Managed with carbamazepine 200 mg in one to two doses or oxcarbazepine 300 mg daily with a max dose of 1200 mg in two dived doses
- If anticonvulsants are not effective use baclofen 15 mg TID with a max of 80 mg per day

## Palliative Care/End of Life Care

- Request a living will before making life-changing decisions for terminally ill patients

# Pediatrics

## Acute Lymphocytic Leukemia (ALL)

- Typically affects children age 6 or younger
- Diagnosed by bone marrow biopsy
- Patient presents with fatigue, easy bruising, fever, dizziness, and shortness of breath
- On exam you should feel lymphadenopathy, enlarged spleen and liver, patient will have pallor with ecchymosis
- Obtain a CBC with diff, CMP, peripheral smear and LD; you should see **anemia with leukocytosis** or leukopenia on your CBC or thrombocytopenia; many patients will have severe neutropenia as well
- Definitely refer

## ADHD

- Hyperactivity and inattention with or without impulsivity
- **Neurological disorder**
- Patient will exhibit symptoms at home and at school; use multiple sources to confirm behavior
- Clinically diagnosed
- **Stimulants considered the number one choice for treatment;** screen children for cardiovascular disease before starting stimulants

## Asthma

- Reactive airway disease, airway obstruction, and airway hyper-responsiveness
- Increased risk if there is a family history, active tobacco smoke exposure, h/o viral infections, allergies, and eczema
- Patient presents with cough especially at night time, expiratory wheezing, shortness of breath, may have atopic disease and wheezing triggered by environmental exposures or emotions
- **Diagnosed with spirometry**; should show that airway disease is reversible after patient receives bronchodilators
- Children aged 0–4: Step 1 use a SAB2A for intermittent and exercise induced asthma; Step 2 is managed with a SAB2A plus low dose ICS or montelukast as an alternative to the ICS; Step 3 requires medium dose ICS and SAB2A; Step 4 is the same as Step 3 plus montelukast; Step 5 requires high-dose ICS plus montelukast and SAB2A; step 6 is the same as Step 5 plus oral corticosteroid
- Children aged 5–11: Step 1, use an SAB2A for intermittent and exercise induced asthma; Step 2 is managed with a SAB2A plus low-dose ICS or montelukast as an alternative to the ICS; Step 3 requires medium-dose ICS and SAB2A or low-dose ICS with a LAB2A or LTRA or theophylline; Step 4, use medium-dose ICS with a LAB2A or LTRA or theophylline; Step 5 requires high-dose ICS with LAB2A or LTRA or theophylline plus SAB2A; Step 6 is the same as Step 5 plus oral corticosteroid
- Children ages 12 and up: Step 1, use an SAB2A for intermittent and exercise-induced asthma; Step 2 is managed with a SAB2A plus low-dose ICS or LTRA or cromolyn or nedocromil or theophylline; Step 3 requires medium-dose ICS and SAB2A or low-dose ICS with a

LAB2A or LTRA or theophylline; Step 4, use medium-dose ICS with a LAB2A or LTRA or theophylline; Step 5 requires high-dose ICS with LAB2A or LTRA or theophylline plus SAB2A and inhaled tiotropium; Step 6 is the same as Step 5 plus oral corticosteroid

## Cephalohematoma

- Hemorrhage of blood that occurs between the skull and periosteum
- During birth, this occurs secondary to a prolonged second stage of labor or from different instruments used in the delivery
- In severe cases, infant presents with jaundice, anemia, and hypotension
- **Infant will have hyperbilirubinemia**

**What to know for the exam:** This is a cause of hyperbilirubinemia at delivery.

## Croup

- Patient presents with a seal-like barky cough
- Must r/o airway obstruction
- Clinically diagnosed but certainly order an x-ray of the neck anteriorly and lateral
- **Steeples sign** will be positive
- Occurs in children age 6 months old to 6 years old
- Treated with oral dexamethasone 0.15mg to 0.6mg/kg x 1 and budesonide inhaled 2mg x 1 with supportive care in moderate cases

**What to know for the exam:** Steeples sign will be positive and the patient's presentation. Do not use long-acting beta 2 to treat CROUP.

## Down Syndrome

- Most common genetic cause of cognitive disability
- Also known as trisomy 21
- Patient is more prone to hearing loss, cognitive disability, delayed speech, delay in gross motor skill development, congenital heart disease, visual abnormalities and hypotonia

**What to know for the exam:** Infant risks, as noted above.

## Epiglottis

- Cellulitis of the supraglottis
- Medical emergency
- Child presents with drooling, high fevers, muffled voice, difficulty breathing, and stridor
- **Positive thumb sign with lateral neck radiograph**
- Management includes intubation or airway protection, IV cefotaxime, racemic epinephrine, and corticosteroids

## Eye Exams for Newborns

- First two months eyes can appear to be crossed
- Subconjunctival hemorrhage common at delivery
- Vision 20/400
- Absent red reflex could be congenital cataract
- White reflex r/o retinoblastoma

## Febrile Seizures

- Divided into three types: simple, complex, and symptomatic
- MMR induced fevers can occur one to two weeks after the injection
- Typically occurs age 6 months to 5 years old with a temp > 100.4
- Seizures are either generalized clonic or tonic-clonic
- Treat underlying cause of fever

**What to know for the exam:** Antipyretics will not prevent febrile seizures. Know that fevers lower a patient's seizure threshold.

## GERD (Infant)

- Think of a child <1 years old with symptoms of regurgitation, abdominal pain, vomiting, etc., within 30 minutes of eating.
- Diagnostic tools include esophageal 24-hour pH study, upper GI contrast study, abdominal x-ray, or abdominal ultrasound
- Rule out food allergies such as diary and gluten
- Switch to thick food or anti-regurgitate formulas and ensure infant is sitting up right during meals

## Gynecomastia

- Can occur unilaterally or bilaterally; 99% of the time this is a benign finding
- Can result from excess estrogen or if a patient has low levels of testosterone
- Can occur in infants, puberty and obesity
- In adolescents, this typically resolves in two years on its own
- Can use estrogen blockers or surgery for persistent cases

**What to know for the exam:** Watch and wait in adolescents; check prolactin level.

## Hydrocele

- Collection of fluid in the tunica vaginalis or the membrane that surrounds the testis
- Common in newborns; generally resolves on its own in a year or two
- If the child is less than 2 years old and not in pain, observation is recommended

**What to know for the exam:** This is common and will spontaneously disappear on its own in a year or two.

## Immunization Tips

- Know that TDAP vaccines are given every 10 years
- Know DTAP stops at age 7
- Know the frequency between giving live viruses
- **Infants born to hepatitis-B-positive mothers need to receive the hepatitis B vaccine and immunoglobulin in the first 12 hours of life.**

## Intussusception

- Infant presents with colicky abdominal pain with **currant jelly stools**; infants have yellow emesis with red stool
- Caused from a prolapse of part of the intestine
- Most commonly occurs in infants age 6 to 12 months and usually happens in male gender
- Order an abdominal plain film x-ray and abdominal ultrasound
- If CT scan ordered there will be a positive "target sign"

- Treat with fluid resuscitation and contrast enema reduction

## Miscellaneous

- Start BP screening at 3 years old
- Never feed an infant goat or cow milk before age 1 year old, as it can cause anemia
- Consider absent seizures in children with blank stares
- Cow's milk leads to anemia because it has less iron then breast milk or formula fortified with iron; it also causes small amounts of blood to be lost though the gut; **check CBC if you suspect anemia in an infant over 8 months, as his or her iron stores from birth will be depleted by then**
- Colic diagnosed by rule of threes: three hours of crying; more than three days a week; symptoms ongoing for at least 3 weeks
- Poisoning is the number one cause of mortality in children
- MVA number one cause of mortality in young adults
- To assess for dehydration in infants check for the presents of tears, their fontanels, skin turgor, and mucous membranes.
- Infant intoeing (metatarsus adductus) is considered benign and will usually disappear after two to three years after birth spontaneously
- Posterior fontanelle's close at two to three months and anterior fontanelles close between six to 18 months

## Morton's Neuroma

- Patient presents with pain in the ball of feet usually between third and fourth toes
- Patient may state it feels like walking on a pebble
- Increased occurrence in ballerinas and people wearing high-heeled shoes
- Treatment is to reduce pressure from around the nerve; arch support and foot pads are helpful; steroid injections are given; in severe cases, decompression surgery is performed

## Osgood–Schlatter Disease

- Always on the exam
- Typical presentation is an adolescent male sports player that comes in with c/o unilateral anterior knee pain; pain is worse with activity
- You palpate and see prominent tibial tubercle, which will be tender to touch
- Treatment includes limiting sports activities, using a compressive bandage and NSAIDS

## Pyloric Stenosis

- Infant presents with emesis after each feeding, which has been ongoing despite changing formula
- Non-bilious projectile vomiting
- **Upper-abdominal olive-shaped mass**
- Can be mistaken for over feeding or GERD
- Treated with IV fluids and surgery

**What to know for the exam:** Remember that infant presents with projectile vomiting with an olive-shaped mass in the right-upper abdomen.

## Rotavirus

- Typically affects children < 5 years old; child presents with vomiting and diarrhea with or without fever
- Dehydration is a serious complication and can lead to metabolic acidosis
- Prevented by immunizations and breast feeding
- Greater risk for children in day care; higher occurrence in the winter months; increased risk in those with immunodeficiency

**What to know for the exam:** Risk factors and presentation.

## Respiratory Syncytial Virus Infection (RSV)

- Most common cause of bronchiolitis; typically occurs in children and older adults
- Child presents with cough, runny nose, wheezing, and respiratory distress
- Treatment is supportive with nasal and pulmonary toilet, oxygen as needed, and nebulized hypertonic saline
- Consider using ribavirin for immunocompromised patient or those with moderate disease

## Talipes Equinovarus (Club Foot)

- Common birth defect
- Patient born with hind foot in varus and the forefoot adducted and ankle is in equinus (upward bending motion)
- Etiology is unknown but is more common in patients with a family history
- Initially treated with manipulation and casting performed by a pediatric orthopedic surgeon

  **What to know for the exam:** Know this from Metatarsus adductus, which presents with the forefoot adducted, but the patient's heel is neutral or just slightly valgus without equinus.

# Respiratory Disorders

## COPD

- Emphysema and chronic bronchitis; occurs when airflow is limited, and the limitation is **not fully reversible**
- Patient may present with a barrel chest, wheezing, tachypnea, cough, and dyspnea
- On exam, listen for hyper-resonance on percussion
- First test to order is spirometry; also obtain a pulse ox
- Consider a chest x-ray which would show hyperinflation
- **Anticholinergics such as tiotropium inhaled drug of choice**
- **Always use SAB2A for rescue and anticholinergics for long-term treatment**

## Pertussis

- Caused by Bordetella pertussis
- Known as the "100-day cough"
- Patient presents with rhinorrhea, fever, sneezing, and mild cough in the catarrhal stage, which lasts for one to two weeks
- In the paroxysmal stage, the cough becomes more severe and persist for two to three weeks, then severity decreases; patients generally have inspiratory whooping cough with emesis; this is the stage when pertussis is usually diagnosed
- In the convalescent stage, the patient's symptoms weaken and disappear after two to three weeks
- Risk factors include infants < 6 months, patients who have not been immunized, school and healthcare workers, and close contact with infected persons

- Obtain a nasopharyngeal culture from the posterior nasopharynx
- Managed with azithromycin in an infant < 1 month old, a macrolide or Bactrim DS in anyone > 1 month old and nonpregnant, and use erythromycin in pregnancy

## Pneumonia

- CAP acquired outside of the hospital
- Clinically diagnosed
- Chest x-ray shows infiltrates
- Patient presents with dyspnea, fever or chills, chest pain, cough with sputum production; usually febrile with myalgia
- Exam findings reveal dullness to percussion of the affected lobe
- **Treat outpatient with macrolides** or tetracyclines first-line therapy
- Patients with comorbidities such as diabetes use a fluoroquinolone
- Repeat chest x-rays after antibiotics therapy is a good way to monitor the patient
- Have patient contact you if his or her symptoms have not improved in 72 hours

**What to know for the exam:** What pneumonia looks like on an x-ray and treatment.

## Pulmonary Embolism (PE)

- Typically occurs in patients who are in a hypercoagulable state (cancer)
- Patient presents with chest pain, shortness of breath, increase work of breathing, and may or may not have syncope
- Patients may have a feeling of impending doom with cough, fever, and tachycardia

- **Increased risk in those with a h/o DVTs, prolonged best rest, recent surgery, cancer patients, pregnant, and elderly**
- **Order a computed tomographic pulmonary angiography of the chest (CTPA), which is 96% sensitive for PEs**
- **Also order a ventilation-perfusion scan (V/Q scan)**
- Life-threatening emergency that is managed inpatient

**What to know for the exam:** Remember patients who are at risk for this and the imaging that you would order.

# Rheumatology

## Systemic Lupus Erythematosus (SLE)

- Chronic autoimmune disorder; can affect multiple systems such as the skin, joints, and kidneys
- Typically affects women during reproductive years
- Patient may present with malar rash "butterfly rash," which covers his or her cheeks and bridge of their nose; rash should not cover nasolabial folds; patient may also have a discoid rash; may c/o fatigue, weight loss, fever, mouth ulcers, joint pain, lymphadenopathy, and more
- **Draw an ANA, ESR, CRP, Smith antigen, dsDNA, CBC, and CMP**
- Management consists of NSAIDS and methotrexate plus folic acid

**What to know for the exam:** Patient will have a positive ANA with SLE.

# Women's Health

## Breast Disorders

- **Fibrocystic breast disease** presents with c/o "lumpy" breast tissue with pain and tenderness that generally occurs around a patient's menses. Order a mammogram and breast ultrasound.
- **Breast biopsies distinguish between breast cancer and fibroids.** Have patient restrict caffeine and sodium in her diet. Use acetaminophen and or ibuprofen for pain.
- Breast Cancer-screening should start at aged 40 until aged 75 for average risk women according to the American Cancer Society guidelines.
- Patient presents with a painless lump noted on exam. The mass is usually fixed and firm. Nipple discharge and skin retractions may be noted.
- **Breast cancer is the most common cancer in American women next to skin cancer.**
- **Aging women typically replace breast tissue with fatty tissue.**
- **Mastitis typically affects lactating women but can affect infants and adolescent girls. Staphylococcus aureus** is the usual suspect that causes this infection. Patient presents with flu-like symptoms, fever, breast pain that is unilateral with warmth to affected breast with red streaks. Advise patient to continue to breast feed eight to 12 times a day and use massage, warm compresses and acetaminophen and or ibuprofen as needed. **Treat with dicloxacillin 250 mg – 500 mg QID. Use Bactrim DS for MRSA related cases.**

## Cervical Cancer

- Fourth most-leading cause of cancer in women worldwide.
- **Risk factors include HPV infection, women aged 40–49, HIV infection, young age at onset of sexual activity, multiple sex partners, and tobacco abuse**
- Patient may present with abnormal vaginal bleeding, bleeding after sex, pelvic pain, cervical mass, and painful sex
- Perform vaginal exam, pap smear, HPV testing, cervical biopsy, or colposcopy
- Treatment depends on staging

**What to know for the exam:** Risk factors.

## Contraceptives

- Progesterone-only pills are recommended for women who smoke and are over the age of 35 years
- Progesterone-only OCP recommended for breast-feeding mothers
- The mini pill (progesterone only oral contraceptive) must be taken the same time each day; if missed by more than three hours, the patient needs to use a backup method for one week
- Estrogen/progestin contraceptives effectively suppress ovulation to prevent pregnancy; comes in pills, patches, and a vaginal ring
- Give higher-dose estrogen combinations for women on anticonvulsants such as phenytoin and carbamazepine
- Women can start COCP regardless of where they are in their menstrual cycle
- Avoid estrogen containing contraceptives in women with multiple cardiovascular risks
- Estrogen OCP are contraindicated in women >35 years old who have migraines with or without aura
- Do not give estrogen OCP pills to women with migraines with aura
- Do not give estrogen OCP to women >35 years old or heavy smokers
- **Advise patient that side effects such as nausea and spotting will typical disappear the first two to three months of contraceptive use**
- Women do not need a pelvic exam before starting them on birth control
- **Plan B (Levonorgestrel):** Emergency contraceptive; give 1.5 mg PO x 1 asap after unprotected intercourse; most effective within 72 hours

of intercourse; must repeat the dose if patient vomits three hours after taking

## Fundal Height

- 12 weeks = symphysis pubis
- 20 weeks = umbilicus
- 36 weeks = xiphoid process

## Infertility

- Risk factors such as PCOS symptoms of hirsutism, acne, and irregular menstrual cycles
- First test ordered semen analysis
- Obtain basal FSH, LH, estradiol, TSH, prolactin, luteal phase progesterone, and transvaginal ultrasound
- **Primary cause worldwide is tubal disease from pelvic infections**
- Although PCOS is thought to be the most common cause, it only occurs in 5% of the population, so keep that in mind

## Miscellaneous

- You cannot give an MMR while a patient is pregnant; wait until after delivery
- Lung cancer kills more women than breast cancer

## Ovarian Cancer

- Patient presents with vague symptoms of abdominal bloating and discomfort, indigestion, pelvic pain, low back pain, and urinary urgency.
- Symptoms have been ongoing for more than three months
- Exam findings will demonstrate a palpable pelvic mass
- **First test ordered is a pelvic ultrasound**
- Biopsies are not recommended routinely; surgery is usually required to adequately diagnose ovarian cancer

## Pap Smear Testing

- Screening starts at age 21 years old; screen once every three years with cytology testing **without** HPV for women with average risk
- Women aged 21–24 years old who are positive for ASC-US or LSIL pap test should be repeated in 12 months
- If a woman is >25 years old and has ASC-US, either repeat pap test in 12 months or add reflex HPV testing
- If a woman is positive for ASC-US cytology and negative for HPV you need to repeat HPV and pap in three years
- If the pap reads normal cytology but absent endocervical cells, you do NOT need to repeat pap test
- Women who are positive for HPV genotype of 16 or 18 should have a colposcopy right away
- Women with average risk and are > 30 years should be screen once every five years with cytology and HPV testing
- Routine HPV screening in women with average risk that are < 30 years old is not recommended
- Women who are positive for ASC-US or higher and are positive for HPV should be referred for a colposcopy; if the woman is positive for ASC-US and negative for HPV, screen her yearly
- Screen women with partial hysterectomies, as they still have their cervix
- Women with complete hysterectomies do not need pap test but still require pelvic exams years; only perform pap test if hysterectomy was for cervical cancer
- Stop performing pap test at age 70 years old if the patient has been having normal test the past 10 years; however, she still requires yearly pelvic exams

## Polycystic Ovarian Syndrome (PCOS)

- A syndrome that causes anovulation, irregular menstrual cycles and issues with fertility
- Patient presents with c/o hirsutism, infertility, abnormal menstrual cycles, acne, and weight gain
- Check FSH, LH, beta HCG, free and total testosterone, TSH, DHEA-S, insulin, prolactin fasting lipids, and fasting glucose; expect patient to have high testosterone and or DHEA with insulin resistant and dyslipidemia
- Advise patients who are wishing to conceive to lose weight as their first line treatment; if weight loss fails to return ovulation, then start patient on metformin to restore ovulation, but it may take six to nine months
- OCP that contain estrogen and progestin block gonadotropin secretion, which will decrease free testosterone

**What to know for the exam:** Patient presentation and the labs you need to draw.

## Placenta Abruption

- This is a premature separation of the placenta from the uterine wall
- Can be total or partial
- Patient has **painful vaginal bleeding**, abdominal pain, uterine contractions, and a tender uterus
- You would order fetal monitor, CBC, coagulation studies, and an ultrasound
- Refer out

**What to know for the exam:** Patient presentation.

## Placenta Previa

- **Can be complete, partial, marginal, or low lying**
- **Occurs when the placenta is literally over the cervical os**
- Patient will present with **painless bright red vaginal bleeding** in the second trimester
- Ultrasound is diagnostic

**What to know for the exam:** Patient presentation.

## Preeclampsia

- HTN in pregnancy that typically occurs after 20 weeks of gestation
- Patient presents with **BP > 140/90, edematous, protein in their urine, elevated LFTs**, headache, and abdominal pain; patient may or may not have low platelets
- Managed by hospital admission with close monitoring of the mother and the baby; delivery is the final treatment; patients with a systolic BP >160 and or a diastolic >110 can be treated with labetalol, nifedipine, hydralazine, or methyldopa

## Primary Amenorrhea

- Patient with either absence of menses by age **13 years old** with no other signs of puberty or patient with secondary sex characteristics but still no menses by age **15 years old**
- Check FSH, serum HCG, LH, TSH, prolactin, DHEA-S, serum estradiol, testosterone, and karyotyping when appropriate
- Variety of causes such as emotional stress, malnutrition, prolactinemia, PCOS, and genetic disorders such as Turner syndrome

## Secondary Amenorrhea

- Occurs in females who have had at least three normal cycles and are currently lacking a cycle in the past six months
- First test to order is an HCG regardless of if the patient says she is sexually active or not
- Check FSH, serum HCG, LH, TSH, prolactin, DHEAS, serum estradiol, and testosterone

# References

1. Aberg JA, Gallant JE, Ghanem KG, et al. Primary care guidelines for the management of persons infected with HIV: 2013 update by the HIV Medicine Association of the Infectious Diseases Society of America. Clinton Infect Dis. 2014;58:e1-e34

2. Abraham P, Avenel A, Park CM, et al. A systematic review of drug therapy for Graves' hyperthyroidism. European J Endocrinol. 2005;153:489-498.

3. Age-Related Eye Disease Study Research Group. A randomized, placebo-controlled, clinical trial of high-dose supplementation with vitamins C and E, beta carotene, and zinc for age-related macular degeneration and vision loss: AREDS report no. 8. Arch Ophthalmology. 2001;119:1417-1436

4. American Academy of Nurse Practitioners (AANP). www.aanp.org

5. American Academy of Ophthalmology. Preferred practice patterns: Conjunctivitis. October 2013. http://one.aao.org (last accessed 30 November 2016)

6. American Academy of Orthopaedic Surgeons. Management of carpal tunnel syndrome evidence-based clinical practice guideline. Feb 2016. http://www.aaos.org

7. American Association of Clinical Endocrinologists; American Thyroid Association. Clinical practice guidelines for hypothyroidism in adults: cosponsored by the American Association of Clinical Endocrinologists and the American Thyroid Association. 2012. http://www.aace.com (last accessed 18 May 2017)

8. American College of Obstetricians and Gynecologists; Task Force on Hypertension in Pregnancy. Hypertension in pregnancy: report of the

American College of Obstetricians and Gynecologists' Task Force on Hypertension in Pregnancy. Obstetric Gynecol. 2013;122:1122-1131.

9. American College of Radiology. ACR appropriateness criteria: left lower quadrant pain - suspected diverticulitis. 2014. http://www.acr.org

10. American College of Radiology. ACR practice parameter for the performance of screening and diagnostic mammography. 2014. http://www.acr.org/

11. American Diabetes Association. Standards of medical care in diabetes - 2017. Diabetes Care. 2017;40 (supplemental 1):S1-S135.

12. American Nurses Credentialing Center. (ANCC). http://www.nursecredentialing.org/

13. American Psychiatric Association. Diagnostic and statistical manual of mental disorders, 5th ed., (DSM-5). Washington, DC: American Psychiatric Publishing; 2013.

14. Andersen JC, Bundgaard L, Elbrønd H, et al. Danish national guidelines for treatment of diverticular disease. Dan Med J. 2012;59:C4453.

15. Anderson J, Caplan L, Yazdany J, et al. Rheumatoid arthritis disease activity measures: American College of Rheumatology recommendations for use in clinical practice. Arthritis Care Res (Hoboken). 2012;64:640-647

16. Aronson JK, Ferner RE. Joining the DoTS: New approach to classifying adverse drug reactions. BMJ. 2003;327:1222-1225

17. Aspelund G, Langer JC. Current management of hypertrophic pyloric stenosis. Semin Pediatr Surg. 2007;16:27-33

18. Atkinson AB, Kennedy A, Wiggam MI, et al. Long-term remission rates after pituitary surgery for Cushing's disease: The need for long-term surveillance. Clin Endocrinol (Oxf). 2005;63:549-559.

19. Baddour LM, Wilson WR, Bayer AS, et al. Infective endocarditis in adults: diagnosis, antimicrobial therapy, and management of complications: a scientific statement for healthcare professionals from the American Heart Association. Circulation. 2015;132:1435-1486.

20. Bedenis R, Stewart M, Cleanthis M, et al. Cilostazol for intermittent claudication. Cochrane Database System Rev. 2014;(10):CD003748.

21. Benito-Leon J, Louis ED. Clinical update: diagnosis and treatment of essential tremor. Lancet. 2007;369:1152-1154

22. Bertsias GK, Ioannidis JPA, Aringer M, et al. EULAR recommendations for the management of systemic lupus erythematosus with neuropsychiatric manifestations: report of a task force of the EULAR standing committee for clinical affairs. Ann Rheum Dis. 2010;69:2074-2082.

23. Betti R, Menni S, Radaelli G, et al. Micronodular basal cell carcinoma: a distinct subtype? Relationship with nodular and infiltrative basal cell carcinomas. J Dermatol. 2010;37:611-616

24. Bickley, Lynn S. (2003). Bates' Guide to Physical Examination and History Taking. Philadelphia: Lippincott. p. 347.

25. Biggs HM, Behravesh CB, Bradley KK, et al. Diagnosis and management of tickborne rickettsial diseases: Rocky Mountain spotted fever and other spotted fever group rickettsioses, ehrlichioses, and anaplasmosis - United States. MMWR Recomm Rep. 2016;65:1-44

26. Branch-Elliman W, Golen TH, Gold HS, et al. Risk factors for Staphylococcus aureus postpartum breast abscess. Clin Infect Dis. 2012;54:71-77

27. Brazzelli M, Cruickshank M, Kilonzo M, et al. Clinical effectiveness and cost-effectiveness of cholecystectomy compared with observation/conservative management for preventing recurrent symptoms and complications in adults presenting with uncomplicated symptomatic gallstones or cholecystitis: a systematic review and economic evaluation. Health Technol Assess. 2014;18:1101

28. Burstein R, Noseda R, Borsook D. Migraine: Multiple processes, complex pathophysiology. J Neurosci. 2015;35:6619-6629

29. Byer NE. Subclinical retinal detachment resulting from asymptomatic retinal breaks: Prognosis for progression and regression. Ophthalmology. 2001;108:1499-1503

30. Caronia LM, Martin C, Welt CK, et al. A genetic basis for functional hypothalamic amenorrhea. N Engl J Med. 2011;364:215-225.

31. Centers for Disease Control and Prevention (CDC) Advisory Committee on Immunization Practices (ACIP). Recommended adult immunization schedule: United States - 2017. February 2017.

32. Centers for Disease Control and Prevention. Laboratory testing for the diagnosis of HIV infection: updated recommendations. June 2014. http://stacks.cdc.gov/

33. Centers for Disease Control and Prevention. Rubella (German measles): 2010 case definition. May 2014. http://www.cdc.gov (last accessed 27 February 2017)

34. Centers for Disease Control and Prevention. Sexually transmitted disease surveillance, 2014. November 2015. http://www.cdc.gov/

35. Charmandari E, Nicolaides NC, Chrousos GP. Adrenal insufficiency. Lancet. 2014;383:2152-2167

36. Chaudhuri A, Martinez-Martin P, Kennedy PG, et al. EFNS Task Force. EFNS guideline on the management of community-acquired bacterial meningitis: report of an EFNS Task Force on acute bacterial

meningitis in older children and adults. Eur J Neurol. 2008;15:649-659. [Erratum in: Eur J Neurol. 2008;15:880.]

37. Chen E, Hornig S, Shepherd SM, et al. Primary closure of mammalian bites. Acad Emerg Med. 2000;7:157-161.

38. Clark GW, Pope SM, Jaboori KA. Diagnosis and treatment of seborrheic dermatitis. Am Fam Physician. 2015;91:185-190

39. Crum RM, Anthony JC, Bassett SS, Folstein MF. Population-based norms for the mini-mental state examination by age and educational level. JAMA. 1993;269(18):2386-2391.

40. Dasgupta B, Borg FA, Hassan N, et al. BSR and BHPR guidelines for the management of giant cell arteritis. Rheumatology (Oxford). 2010;49:1594-1597.

41. Dean B, Becker G, Little C. The management of the acute traumatic subungual haematoma: A systematic review. Hand Surg. 2012. 17(1):151-4.

42. Deschenes J, Murray PI, Rao NA, et al.; International Uveitis Study Group. International Uveitis Study Group (IUSG): Clinical classification of uveitis. Ocul Immunol Inflamm. 2008;16:1-2

43. Devalia V, Hamilton MS, Molloy AM; British Committee for Standards in Haematology. Guidelines for the diagnosis and treatment of cobalamin and folate disorders. Br J Haematol. 2014;166:496-513.

44. Dolin R. Hand-foot-and-mouth disease. In: Freedberg I, ed. Fitzpatrick's dermatology in general medicine. 6th ed. New York, NY: McGraw-Hill; 2003:2049-2052

45. Dowman JK, Tomlinson JW, Newsome PN. Systematic review: the diagnosis and staging of non-alcoholic fatty liver disease and non-alcoholic steatohepatitis. Aliment Pharmacol Ther. 2011;33:525-540

46. Drake LA, Dinehart SM, Farmer ER, et al. Guidelines of care for superficial mycotic infections of the skin: tinea corporis, tinea cruris, tinea faciei, tinea manuum, and tinea pedis. Guidelines/Outcomes Committee. American Academy of Dermatology. J Am Acad Dermatol. 1996;34:282-286

47. Elwood JM, Jospson J. Melanoma and sun exposure: an overview of published studies. Int J Cancer. 1997;73:198-203

48. Epocrates [online]. San Francisco, CA: Epocrates, Inc.; 2013. http://www.epocrates.com. Updated continuously. Accessed Novermber, 15, 2017.

49. Erb KJ (2007). "Helminths, allergic disorders and IgE-mediated immune responses: where do we stand?" Eur. J. Immunol. 37(5): 1170–3. PMID 17447233. doi:10.1002/eji.200737314

50. Eriksson B, Jorup-Ronstrom C, Karkkonen K, et al. Erysipelas: clinical and bacteriologic spectrum and serological aspects. Clin Infect Dis. 1996;23:1091-1098

51. Evers S, Jensen R, European Federation of Neurological Societies. Treatment of medication overuse headache - guideline of the EFNS headache panel. Eur J Neurol. 2011;18:1115-1121

52. Fleming GF, Ronette BM, Seidman J, et al. Epithelial ovarian cancer. In: Barakat RR, Markman M, Randall ME, eds. Principles and practice of gynecologic oncology. 5th ed. Philadelphia, PA: Lippincott, Williams & Wilkins; 2009.

53. Forbes TJ, Kim DW, Du W, et al; CCISC Investigators. Comparison of surgical, stent, and balloon angioplasty treatment of native coarctation of the aorta: An observational study by the CCISC (Congenital Cardiovascular Interventional Study Consortium). J Am Coll Cardiol. 2011;58:2664-2674

54. Forcier M, Musacchio N. An overview of human papillomavirus infection for the dermatologist: disease, diagnosis, management, and prevention. Dermatol Ther. 2010;23:458-476.
55. Francis GJ, Becker WJ, Pringsheim TM. Acute and preventive pharmacologic treatment of cluster headache. Neurology. 2010;75:463-473.
56. Frobell RB, Roos EM, Roos HP, et al. A randomized trial of treatment for acute anterior cruciate ligament tears. N Engl J Med. 2010;363:331-342. [Erratum in: N Engl J Med. 2010;363:893
57. Gaffield ME, Culwell KR, Lee CR. The use of hormonal contraception among women taking anticonvulsant therapy. Contraception. 2011;83:16-29
58. Gholve PA, Scher DM, Khakharia S, et al. Osgood Schlatter syndrome. Curr Opin Pediatr. 2007;19:44-50.
59. Global Initiative for Asthma. Pocket guide for asthma management and prevention for children 5 years and younger. 2015. http://www.ginasthma.org/ (last accessed 18 August 2016).
60. Global Initiative for Chronic Obstructive Lung Disease (GOLD). GOLD 2017 global strategy for the diagnosis, management, and prevention of chronic obstructive pulmonary disease. 2017. http://www.goldcopd.org/ (last accessed 12 May 2017)
61. Gupta AK, Paquet M, Villanueva E, et al. Interventions for actinic keratoses. Cochrane Database Syst Rev. 2012;(12):CD004415
62. Gupta K, Hooton TM, Naber KG, et al. International clinical practice guidelines for the treatment of acute uncomplicated cystitis and pyelonephritis in women: a 2010 update by the Infectious Diseases Society of America and the European Society for Microbiology and Infectious Diseases. Clin Infect Dis. 2011;52:e103-120

63. Habib G, Lancellotti P, Antunes MJ, et al. 2015 ESC Guidelines for the management of infective endocarditis. Eur Heart J. 2015;36:3075-3128

64. Hall CD, Weinberg GA, Iwane MK, et al. The burden of respiratory syncytial virus infection in young children. N Engl J Med. 2009'360: 588-598

65. Hendricks KA, Wright ME, Shadomy SV, et al. Centers for Disease Control and Prevention expert panel meetings on preventions and treatment of anthrax in adults. Emerg Infect Dis 2014;20.

65. Henton J, Jain A. Cochrane corner: antibiotic prophylaxis for mammalian bites (intervention review). J Hand Surg Eur Vol. 2012;37:804-806

66. Higgs DR, Engel JD, Stamatoyannopoulos G. Thalassaemia. Lancet. 2012;379:373-383

67. Hoelzer D, Gökbuget N, Ottmann O, et al. Acute lymphoblastic leukemia. Hematology Am Soc Hematol Educ Prog. 2002:162-192

68. Hu T, Mills KT, Yao L, et al. Effects of low-carbohydrate diets versus low-fat diets on metabolic risk factors: a meta-analysis of randomized controlled clinical trials. Am J Epidemiol. 2012;176(suppl 7):S44-S54.

69. Huang JQ, Sridhar S, Hunt RH. Role of Helicobacter pylori infection and nonsteroidal anti-inflammatory drugs in peptic-ulcer disease: a meta-analysis. Lancet. 2002;359:14-2

70. Lacroix A, Feelders RA, Stratakis CA, et al. Cushing's syndrome. Lancet. 2015;386:913-927

71. Law S, Derry S, Moore RA. Triptans for acute cluster headache. Cochrane Database Syst Rev. 2013:(7);CD008042

72. Lazzaroni M, Bianchi Porro G. Gastrointestinal side-effects of traditional nonsteroidal anti-inflammatory drugs and new formulations. Aliment Pharmacol Ther. 2004;20(suppl 2):48-58

73. Lederman C, Miller M. Hordeola and chalazia. Pediatr Rev. 1999;20:283-284

74. Lieberthal AS, Carroll AE, Chonmaitree T, et al. The diagnosis and management of acute otitis media. Pediatrics. 2013;131:e964-e999

75. Lin JS, Eder M, Weinmann S. Behavioral counseling to prevent skin cancer: a systematic review for the U.S. Preventive Services Task Force. Ann Intern Med. 2011;154:190-201

76. Lindsley K, Matsumura S, Hatef E, Akpek EK. Interventions for chronic blepharitis. Cochrane Database Syst Rev. 2012;5:CD005556

77. Lopez LM, Newmann SJ, Grimes DA, et al. Immediate start of hormonal contraceptives for contraception. Cochrane Database Syst Rev. 2012;(12):CD006260

78. James PA, Oparil S, Carter BL, Cushman WC, Dennison-Himmelfarb C, Handler J, Lackland DT, LeFevre ML, MacKenzie TD, Ogedegbe O, Smith SC, Svetkey LP, Taler SJ, Townsend RR, Wright JT, Narva AS, Ortiz E. 2014 Evidence-Based Guideline for the Management of High Blood Pressure in AdultsReport From the Panel Members Appointed to the Eighth Joint National Committee (JNC 8). JAMA. 2014;311(5):507–520. doi:10.1001/jama.2013.284427

79. January CT, Wann LS, Alpert JS, et al. 2014 AHA/ACC/HRS guideline for the management of patients with atrial fibrillation: a report of the American College of Cardiology/American Heart Association Task Force on Practice Guidelines and the Heart Rhythm Society. J Am Coll Cardiol. 2014;64:e1-e76

80. Jelks A, Cifuentes R, Ross MG (October 2007). "Clinician bias in fundal height measurement". Obstet Gynecol. 110 (4): 892–9

81. Johnson D, Klassen T, Kellner J. Diagnosis and management of croup: Alberta Medical Association clinical practice guidelines. Alberta: Alberta Medical Association; 2015. http://www.topalbertadoctors.org (last accessed 22 October 2016)

82. Johnson NP, Bontekoe S, Stewart AW. Analysis of factors predicting success of metformin and clomiphene treatment for women with infertility owing to PCOS-related ovulation dysfunction in a randomised controlled trial. Aust N Z J Obstet Gynaecol. 2011;51:252-256

83. International Pediatric Endosurgery Group. IPEG guidelines for inguinal hernia and hydrocele. J Laparoendosc Adv Surg Tech A. 2010;20:x-xiv

84. Katz PO, Gerson LB, Vela MF. Guidelines for the diagnosis and management of gastroesophageal reflux disease. Am J Gastroenterol. 2013;108:308-328.

85. Kazlauskaite R, Evans AT, Villabona CV, et al. Corticotropin tests for hypothalamic-pituitary-adrenal insufficiency: a metaanalysis. J Clin Endocrinol Metab. 2008;93:4245-4253

86. Keay L, Lindsley K, Tielsch J, et al. Routine preoperative medical testing for cataract surgery. Cochrane Database Syst Rev. 2012;(3):CD007293

87. Khasnis A, Gokula RM (1 April 2003). "Romberg's test". Journal of Postgraduate Medicine. 49 (2): 169–72. PMID Kliegman RM, Stanton BMD, Geme JS, Schor N, Behrman RE. Nelson Textbook of Pediatrics. 19th ed. Saunders; 2011

88. Koopman L, Hoes AW, Glasziou PP, et al. Antibiotic therapy to prevent the development of asymptomatic middle ear effusion in children with acute otitis media: a meta-analysis of individual patient data. Arch Otolaryngol Head Neck Surg. 2008; 134:128-132.

89. Kyle RA, Rajkumar SV. Multiple myeloma. N Engl J Med. 2004; 351:1860-1873.

90. Lockhart PB, Brennan MT, Sasser HC, et al. Bacteremia associated with toothbrushing and dental extraction. Circulation. 2008;117:3118-3125

91. Mardani-Kivi M, Karimi Mobarakeh M, Bahrami F, et al. Corticosteroid injection with or without thumb spica cast for de Quervain tenosynovitis. J Hand Surg Am. 2014;39:37-41.

92. Maruthur NM, Tseng E, Hutfless S, et al. Diabetes medications as monotherapy or metformin-based combination therapy for type 2 diabetes: a systematic review and meta-analysis. Ann Intern Med. 2016;164:740-751

93. McDermott MM, Liu K, Greenland P, et al. Functional decline in peripheral arterial disease: associations with the ankle brachial index and leg symptoms. JAMA. 2004;292:453-461

94. McKeith IG, Dickson DW, Lowe J, et al. Diagnosis and management of dementia with Lewy bodies: third report of the DLB Consortium. Neurology. 2005;65:1863-1872

95. Melmed S, Casanueva FF, Hoffman AR, et al. Endocrine Society. Diagnosis and treatment of hyperprolactinemia: an Endocrine Society clinical practice guideline. J Clin Endocrinol Metab. 2011;96:273-288.

96. Menter A, Korman NJ, Elmets CA, et al. Guidelines of care for the management of psoriasis and psoriatic arthritis: section 3. Guidelines of care for the management and treatment of psoriasis with topical therapies. J Am Acad Dermatol. 2009;60:643-659.

97. Mcnamara DR, Tleyjeh IM, Berbari EF, et al. Incidence of lower-extremity cellulitis: a population-based study in Olmsted County, Minnesota. Mayo Clin Proc. 2007;82:817-821

98. Miller NR, Newman NJ, et al, eds. Walsh & Hoyt's Clinical Neuro-ophthalmology: The Essentials. 2nd ed. Lippincott Williams & Wilkins; 2008. 122-145.

99. Milne L. Ottawa ankle decision rules. West J Med. 1996;164:67

100. Mohney BG. Common forms of childhood strabismus in an incidence cohort. Am J Ophthalmol. 2007;144:465-467

101. National Comprehensive Cancer Network. Clinical practice guidelines in oncology: breast cancer screening and diagnosis. 2016. http://www.nccn.org/

102. National Comprehensive Cancer Network. Clinical practice guidelines in oncology: prostate cancer. Version 3. 2016. http://www.nccn.org (last accessed 12 September 2016).

103. National Comprehensive Cancer Network. NCCN clinical practice guidelines in oncology: testicular cancer. 2016. http://www.nccn.org/ (last accessed 8 September 2016)

104. National Heart, Lung, and Blood Institute. Evidence-based management of sickle cell disease: expert panel report, 2014. September 2014. http://www.nhlbi.nih.gov/ (last accessed 29 November 2016)

105. National Heart, Lung, and Blood Institute; National Asthma Education and Prevention Prog. Guidelines for the diagnosis and management of asthma. July 2007. http://www.nhlbi.nih.gov/ (last accessed 18 August 2016)

106. National Institute for Health and Care Excellence. Colorectal cancer: the diagnosis and management of colorectal cancer. December 2014. http://guidance.nice.org.uk

107. National Institute for Health and Care Excellence. Hypertension in pregnancy: diagnosis and management. January 2011. http://www.nice.org.uk

108. National Institute for Health and Care Excellence. Prophylaxis against infective endocarditis: antimicrobial prophylaxis against infective endocarditis in adults and children undergoing interventional procedures. July 2016. http://www.nice.org.uk (last accessed 28 November 2016

109. National Institute for Health and Care Excellence. Tuberculosis. May 2016. https://www.nice.org.uk/guidance/ng33

110. Newburger JW, Takahashi M, Gerber MA, et al. Diagnosis, treatment, and long-term management of Kawasaki disease: a statement for health professionals from the Committee on Rheumatic Fever, Endocarditis, and Kawasaki Disease, Council on Cardiovascular Disease in the Young, American Heart Association. Pediatrics. 2004; 114:1708-1733

111. Nickel JC, Teichman JM, Gregoire M, et al. Prevalence, diagnosis, characterization, and treatment of prostatitis, interstitial cystitis, and epididymitis in outpatient urological practice: the Canadian PIE Study. Urology. 2005;66:935-940

112. Nieman LK, Biller BM, Findling JW, et al. Treatment of Cushing's syndrome: An Endocrine Society clinical practice guideline. J Clin Endocrinol Metab. 2015;100:2807-2831.

113. Niewoehner CB, Schorer AE. Gynaecomastia and breast cancer in men. BMJ. 2008;336:709-713

114. Nishimura RA, Otto CM, Bonow RO, et al. 2014 AHA/ACC guideline for the management of patients with valvular heart disease: a report of the American College of Cardiology/American Heart Association Task Force on Practice Guidelines. Circulation. 2014;129:e521-e643

115. Nussbaum R, McInnes R, Willard H, et al. Thompson & Thompson genetics in medicine, 6th ed. Philadelphia, PA: Saunders; 2004:157-179

116. Parker LA. Part 1: early recognition and treatment of birth trauma: injuries to the head and face. Adv Neonatal Care. 2005;5(6):288–97. doi: 10.1016/j.adnc.2005.09.001.

117. Pichler WJ. Drug Hypersensitivity Reactions: Classification and Relationship to T-Cell Activation. In: Drug Hypersensitivity, Pichler WJ (Ed), Karger Publishers, Basel 200

118. Ponikowski P, Voors AA, Anker SD, et al. 2016 ESC Guidelines for the diagnosis and treatment of acute and chronic heart failure: the task force for the diagnosis and treatment of acute and chronic heart failure

of the European Society of Cardiology (ESC). Eur J Heart Fail. 2016;18:891-975.

119. Powell, J. Wilson, An evidence-based review of peritonsillar abscess, Clinical Otolaryngology. 37 (2012) 136–145. doi:10.1111/j.1749-4486.2012.02452.x.

120. Practice Committee of the American Society for Reproductive Medicine. Current evaluation of amenorrhea. Fertil Steril. 2008;90(suppl 3):S219-S225

121. Practice Committee of the American Society of Reproductive Medicine. Definitions of infertility and recurrent pregnancy loss: a committee opinion. Fertil Steril. 2013;99:63

122. Prinzmetal's Angina, "Variant Angina and Angina Inversa". American Heart Association. Retrieved 2015-06-20

123. Pui CH, Relling MV, Downing JR. Acute lymphoblastic leukemia. N Engl J Med. 2004;350:1535-1548.

124. Publications Committee, Society for Maternal-Fetal Medicine, Belfort MA. Placenta accreta. Am J Obstet Gynecol. 2010;203:430-439.

125. Razonable RR, Paya CV. Beta-herpesviruses in transplantation. Rev Med Microbiol. 2002;13:163-176.

126. Ranki A, Hyry H, Klimenko T, et al. Update on current care guidelines. Bacterial skin infections [in Finnish]. Duodecim. 2010;126:2883-2884

127. Ringdahl E, Teague L. Testicular torsion. Am Fam Physician. 2006;74:1739-1743

128. Rivadeneira D E, Steele SR, Ternent C, et al. Practice parameters for the management of hemorrhoids (revised 2010). Dis Colon Rectum. 2011;54:1059-1064.

129. Roland PS, Smith TL, Schwartz SR, et al. Clinical practice guideline: cerumen impaction. Otolaryng Head Neck Surg. 2008;139(suppl 2):S1-S21

130. Rosenfeld RM, Piccirillo JF, Chandrasekhar SS, et al. Clinical practice guideline (update): adult sinusitis. Otolaryngol Head Neck Surg. 2015;152(suppl 2):S1-S39

131. Rosenfeld RM, Schwartz SR, Cannon CR, et al. American Academy of Otolaryngology-Head and Neck Surgery Foundation. Clinical practice guideline: acute otitis externa. Otolaryngol Head Neck Surg. 2014;150(suppl 1):S1-S

132. Sanders DB, Wolfe GI, Benatar M, et al. International consensus guidance for management of myasthenia gravis: executive summary. Neurology. 2016;87:419-425.

133. Santen RJ, Mansel R. Benign breast disorders. N Engl J Med. 2005;353:275-285

134. Seidman MD, Gurgel RK, Lin SY; Guideline Otolaryngology Development Group. AAO-HNSF. Clinical practice guideline: Allergic rhinitis. Otolaryngol Head Neck Surg. 2015;152:S1-43

135. Shaheen NJ, Falk GW, Iyer PG, et al. ACG Clinical Guideline: diagnosis and management of Barrett's esophagus. Am J Gastroenterol. 2016;111:30-50;quiz 51.

136. Sharma L, Kapoor D, Issa S. Epidemiology of osteoarthritis: an update. Curr Opin Rheumatol. 2006;18:147-156

137. Shimohata H, Higuchi T, Ogawa Y, et al. Human parvovirus B19-induced acute glomerulonephritis: a case report. Ren Fail. 2013;35:159-162

138. Shoback DM, Bilezikian JP, Costa AG, et al. Presentation of hypoparathyroidism: etiologies and clinical features. J Clin Endocrinol Metab. 2016;101:2300-2312.

139. Silverberg NB. Warts and molluscum in children. Adv Dermatol. 2004;20:23-73

140. Soubrier M, Dubost JJ, Ristori JM. Polymyalgia rheumatica: diagnosis and treatment. Joint Bone Spine. 2006;73:599-605.

141. Staheli L, ed. Clubfoot: Ponseti management, 3rd ed. Seattle, WA: Global HELP; 2009

142. Stein PD, Fowler SE, Goodman LR, et al. Multidetector computed tomography for acute pulmonary embolism. N Engl J Med. 2006;354:2317-2327

143. Stone NJ, Robinson JG, Lichtenstein AH, et al; American College of Cardiology/American Heart Association Task Force on Practice Guidelines. 2013 ACC/AHA guideline on the treatment of blood cholesterol to reduce atherosclerotic cardiovascular risk in adults: a report of the American College of Cardiology/American Heart Association Task Force on Practice Guidelines. J Am Coll Cardiol. 2014;63(25 patient B):2889-2934

144. Swami A, Spodick DH. Pulsus paradoxus in cardiac tamponade: a pathophysiologic continuum. Clin Cardiol 2003; 26:215. Syphilis. In: Kimberlin DW, Brady MT, eds. Red Book: 2015 report of the Committee on Infectious Diseases. 30th ed. Elk Grove Village, IL: American Academy of Pediatrics; 2015:755-768

145. Sysko R, Sha N, Wang Y, et al. Early response to antidepressant treatment in bulimia nervosa. Psychol. Med. 2010;40:999-1005

146. Terkeltaub R, Furst RE, Bennett K, et al. Colchicine efficacy assessed by time to 50% reduction of pain is comparable in low dose and high dose regimens: secondary analyses of the AGREE trial. Abstract presented at: American College of Rheumatology Scientific Meeting; October 2009; Philadelphia, PA.

147. Terkeltaub R, Schumacher HR Jr, Saag KG, et al. Evaluation of rilonace Patient for prevention of gout flares during initiation of urate-lowering therapy: results of a phase 3, randomized, double-blind, placebo-controlled trial. Arthritis Rheum. 2010;62(suppl):152.

148. Terrault NA, Bzowej NH, Chang KM, et al. AASLD guidelines for treatment of chronic hepatitis B. Hepatology. 2016;63:261-283

149. The PIOPED Investigators. Value of the ventilation/perfusion scan in acute pulmonary embolism. Results of the prospective investigation of

pulmonary embolism diagnosis (PIOPED). JAMA. 1990;263:2753-2759

150. Thiboutot DM, Strauss JS. Diet and acne revisited. Arch Dermatol. 2002;138:1591-1592

151. Thomas KE, Hasbun R, Jekel J, et al. The diagnostic accuracy of Kernig's sign, Brudzinski's sign, and nuchal rigidity in adults with suspected meningitis. Clin Infect Dis. 2002;35:46-52 "tyramine | C8H11NO". PubChem. Retrieved 2017-04-08.

152. Walker, Julia J., & Dave, Shashank J. (2009). "Road Cycling Injuries". In Buschbacher, Ralph M., Prahlow, Nathan D., & Dave, Shashank J., Sports Medicine and Rehabilitation(2nd Edition, p 113). Philadelphia, PA: Lippincott Williams & Wilkins.

153. Walton SF, Currie BJ. Problems in diagnosing scabies, a global disease in human and animal populations. Clin Microbiol Rev. 2007;20:268-279

154. Wang K, Bettiol S, Thompson MJ, et al. Symptomatic treatment of the cough in whooping cough. Cochrane Database Syst Rev. 2014;(9):CD003257

155. Wang QP, Bai M. Topiramate versus carbamazepine for the treatment of classical trigeminal neuralgia: a meta-analysis. CNS Drugs. 2011;25:847-857

156. Watts NB, Adler RA, Bilezikian JP, et al. Osteoporosis in men: an Endocrine Society clinical practice guideline. J Clin Endocrinol Metab. 2012;97:1802-1822

157. Weinstein JN, Tosteson TD, Lurie JD, et al. Surgical versus nonoperative treatment for lumbar spinal stenosis four-year results of the Spine Patient Outcomes Research Trial. Spine (Phila Pa 1976). 2010;35:1329-1338

158. Whitehouse JS, Gourlay DM, Winthrop AL, et al. Is it safe to discharge intussusception patients after successful hydrostatic reduction? J Pediatric Surg. 2010;45:1182-1186

159. Wolfe F, Clauw DJ, Fitzcharles MA, et al. Fibromyalgia criteria and severity scales for clinical and epidemiological studies: a modification of the ACR Preliminary Diagnostic Criteria for Fibromyalgia. J Rheumatol. 2011;38:1113-1122.

160. World Gastroenterology Organisation (WGO). WGO practice guideline: acute diarrhea. 2012. http://www.worldgastroenterology.org/ (last accessed 26 January 2017)

161. World Health Organization. International Agency for Research on Cancer. GLOBOCAN 2012: estimated cancer incidence, mortality and prevalence worldwide in 2012. 2015. http://globocan.iarc.fr/ (last accessed 20 January 2017).

162. World Health Organization. Medical eligibility criteria for contraceptive use. 5th ed. 2015. http://www.who.int

163. Workowski KA, Bolan GA; Centers for Disease Control and Prevention (CDC). Sexually transmitted diseases treatment guidelines, 2015. MMWR Recomm Rep. 2015;64:1-137

164. Viswanathan G, Upadhyay A. Assessment of proteinuria. Adv Chronic Kidney Dis. 2011;18:243-248

165. Weinreb RN, Khaw PT. Primary open-angle glaucoma. Lancet. 2004;363:1711-1720

166. Wilkin J, Dahl M, Detmar M, et al. Standard classification of rosacea: report of the National Rosacea Society Expert Committee on the Classification and Staging of Rosacea. J Am Acad Dermatol. 2002;46:584-58

167. Wilson SA, Last A. Management of corneal abrasions. Am Fam Physician. 2004;70:123-128.

168. Wormser GP, Dattwyler RJ, Shapiro ED, et al. The clinical assessment, treatment, and prevention of Lyme disease, human granulocytic anaplasmosis, and babesiosis: clinical practice guidelines

by the Infectious Diseases Society of America. Clin Infect Dis. 2006;43:1089-1134

169. Yamanishi K, Okuno T, Shiraki K, et al. Identification of human herpesvirus-6 as a causal agent for exanthem subitum. Lancet. 1988;1:1065-1067

170. Yancy CW, Jessup M, Bozkurt B, et al. 2013 ACCF/AHA guideline for the management of heart failure: a report of the American College of Cardiology Foundation/American Heart Association Task Force on Practice Guidelines. Circulation. 2013;128:e240-e319

171. Yanoff, Myron; Duker, Jay S. (2008). Ophthalmology (3rd ed.). Edinburgh: Mosby. pp. 1482–1485

172. Yinon Y, Farine D, Yudin MH, et al; Fetal Medicine Committee, Society of Obstetricians and Gynaecologists of Canada. Cytomegalovirus infection in pregnancy. J Obstet Gynaecol Can. 2010;32:348-354

173. Yoder JS, Gargano JW, Wallace RM, et al; Centers for Disease Control and Prevention (CDC). Giardiasis surveillance - United States, 2009-2010. MMWR Surveill Summ. 2012;61:13-23

## Abbreviations

a.c.: Before meals. As in taking a medicine before meals

a/g ratio: Albumin to globulin ratio

ACEI: Ace inhibitor

ACL: Anterior cruciate ligament

ARB: Angiotensin receptor blockers

ARF: Acute renal failure

ADHD: Attention deficit hyperactivity disorder

AIDS: Acquired immune deficiency syndrome

ANA: Antinuclear antibody

ASC-US: Atypical Squamous cells of undetermined significance

ASCVD: Atherosclerotic cardiovascular disease

ASA: Aspirin

Asap: As soon as possible

BCC: Basal cell carcinoma

BID: Twice a day

BMP: Basic metabolic panel

BNP: B-Type natriuretic peptide

BP: Blood pressure

BV: Bacterial vaginosis

CAD: Coronary artery disease

CAP: Community acquired pneumonia

C&S: Culture and sensitivity

C/O: Complaint of

CBC: Complete blood count

CC: Cubic centimeters

CCB: Calcium channel blocker

CK: Creatine kinase

CKD: Chronic kidney disease

CMV: Cytomegalovirus Infection

COPD: Chronic obstructive pulmonary disease

CVA: Cerebrovascular accident

CVD: Cardiovascular disease

D/C: Discontinue

DHEA-S: Dehydroepiandrosterone

DIP: Distal interphalangeal joint

DJD: Degenerative joint disease

DM: Diabetes mellitus

DVT: Deep venous thrombosis

EMG: Electromyographic

ER: Emergency room

ESR: Erythrocyte sedimentation rate

FH: Family history

FSH: Follicle stimulating hormone

FX: Fracture

GAS: Group A streptococcal

GFR: Glomerular filtration rate

H2: Histamine 2

HCG: Human chorionic gonadotropin

H&P: History and physical examination.

H/O or h/o: History of

HPV: Human papillomavirus

HTN: Hypertension

H.S.: At bedtime

I & D: Incision and drainage

IBD: Inflammatory bowel disease

IM: Intramuscular

IR: Insulin resistance

IV: Intravenous fluid

IVDA: Intravenous drug abuse

LAB2A: Long-acting beta 2 agonist

LFTs: Liver function test

LH: Luteinizing hormone

LLQ: Left lower quadrant

LSIL: Low grade squamous intraepithelial lesions

LTRA: Leukotriene receptor antagonist

LUQ: Left upper quadrant

MCL: Medial collateral ligament

MCP: metacarpal-phalangeal

mg: Milligrams

ml: Milliliters

MRI: Magnetic resonance Imaging

MRSA: Methicillin-resistant Staphylococcus aureus

MVP: Mitral valve prolapse

NSAIDs: Nonsteroidal anti-inflammatory drugs

N/V: Nausea and vomiting

OA: Osteoarthritis

OCP: Oral contraceptive

OP: Osteoporosis

PCL: Posterior cruciate ligament

PCN: Penicillin

PCOS: Polycystic ovarian syndrome

PE: Pulmonary embolism

PO: By mouth

PPD: Purified protein derivative

PPI: Proton-pump inhibitors

Pt: Patient

PT: Prothrombin time

PTT: Partial thromboplastin time

PTH: Parathyroid hormone

PUD: Peptic ulcer disease

q.d.: Each day

q.i.d.: Four times daily

q2h: Every 2 hours

q3h: Every 3 hours

qAM: Each morning

qhs: At each bedtime

qod: Every other day

qPM: Each evening

RA: Rheumatoid arthritis

RF: Rheumatoid factor

R.I.C.E: Rest ice compression and elevation

R/O: Rule out

RLQ: Right lower quadrant

RPR: Rapid plasma antigen

RUQ: Right upper quadrant

SCC: Squamous cell carcinoma

SK: Seborrheic keratosis

SLE: Systemic lupus erythematosus

SNRI: Serotonin and norepinephrine reuptake inhibitors

SOB: Shortness of breath

SSRI: Selective serotonin reuptake inhibitor

STI: Sexually transmitted infection

Strep: Streptococcus

Sub Q: Subcutaneous

t.i.d.: Three times daily

tab: Tablet

TAH: Total abdominal hysterectomy

TCA: Tricyclic antidepressants

TFT: Thyroid function test

TIA: Transient ischemic attack

TSH: Thyroid stimulating hormone

UA or u/a: Urinalysis

URI: Upper respiratory tract infection

UTI: urinary tract infection

VDRL: Venereal disease research laboratory test

Made in the USA
Las Vegas, NV
17 April 2023

70733507R00079